TEXT BOOK OF

HOSPITAL AND CLINICAL PHARMACY

For

Second Year Diploma in Pharmacy

Dr. A. V. YADAV
M. Pharm. LL.B., Ph.D.
Head of Pharmacy Deptt;
Government College of Pharmacy
KARAD.

B. V. YADAV
M. Pharm., D.B.M.
Bharati Vidyapeeth's
Institute of Pharmacy (Polytechnic)
Erandwane, PUNE.

Price ₹ 225.00

NIRALI PRAKASHAN
ADVANCEMENT OF KNOWLEDGE

N1261

Hospital and Clinical Pharmacy ISBN 978-81-85790-26-8

Eleventh Edition : August 2020

Published By :
NIRALI PRAKASHAN
Abhyudaya Pragati, 1312, Shivaji Nagar
Off J.M. Road, Pune – 411005
Tel - (020) 25512336/37/39, Fax - (020) 25511379
Email : niralipune@pragationline.com

(–Ve)

Printed By :
RACHANA OFFSETS
S. No. 15, Arihant Marg,
Sukhsagr Nagar, Katraj
Phone : (020) 2778 2011

➤ DISTRIBUTION CENTRES

PUNE

Nirali Prakashan (For orders within Pune) : 119, Budhwar Peth, Jogeshwari Mandir Lane, Pune 411002, Maharashtra
Tel : (020) 2445 2044, Mobile : 9657703145
Email : niralilocal@pragationline.com

Nirali Prakashan (For orders outside Pune) : S. No. 28/27, Dhayari, Near Asian College Pune 411041
Tel : (020) 24690204 Fax : (020) 24690316; Mobile : 9657703143
Email : bookorder@pragationline.com

MUMBAI

Nirali Prakashan : 385, S.V.P. Road, Rasdhara Co-op. Hsg. Society Ltd.,
Girgaum, Mumbai 400004, Maharashtra; Mobile : 9320129587
Tel : (022) 2385 6339 / 2386 9976, Fax : (022) 2386 9976
Email : niralimumbai@pragationline.com

➤ DISTRIBUTION BRANCHES

JALGAON

Nirali Prakashan : 34, V. V. Golani Market, Navi Peth, Jalgaon 425001, Maharashtra,
Tel : (0257) 222 0395, Mob : 94234 91860; Email : niralijalgaon@pragationline.com

KOLHAPUR

Nirali Prakashan : New Mahadvar Road, Kedar Plaza, 1st Floor Opp. IDBI Bank, Kolhapur 416 012
Maharashtra. Mob : 9850046155; Email : niralikolhapur@pragationline.com

NAGPUR

Nirali Prakashan : Above Maratha Mandir, Shop No. 3, First Floor,
Rani Jhanshi Square, Sitabuldi, Nagpur 440012, Maharashtra
Tel : (0712) 254 7129; Email : niralinagpur@pragationline.com

DELHI

Nirali Prakashan : 4593/15, Basement, Agarwal Lane, Ansari Road, Daryaganj
Near Times of India Building, New Delhi 110002 Mob : 08505972553
Email : niralidelhi@pragationline.com

BENGALURU

Nirali Prakashan : Maitri Ground Floor, Jaya Apartments, No. 99, 6th Cross, 6th Main,
Malleswaram, Bengaluru 560003, Karnataka; Mob : 9449043034
Email: niralibangalore@pragationline.com

Other Branches : Hyderabad, Chennai

niralipune@pragationline.com | www.pragationline.com
Also find us on f www.facebook.com/niralibooks

Preface ...

With the implementation of new Education Regulations (ER - 91), Diploma in Pharmacy is gradually getting a clinical orientation. The opportunity to prepare a new book on "Hospital and Clinical Pharmacy" provided us the occasion to serve to the students of Diploma course in Pharmacy.

We take pleasure in presenting this book to provide the students updated and collective information on various aspects of Hospital and Clinical Pharmacy in a simple and lucid language.

We sincerely hope that the students and staff will appreciate our efforts and provide us with necessary feed-back to make essential improvements in the book.

We are thankful to the Publisher Shri. Dineshbhai Furia and Shri. Jignesh Furia for bringing out the book in nice form.

Authors

Syllabus ...

PART - I : HOSPITAL PHARMACY

1. **Hospitals:** Definition, Function, Classifications based on various criteria, Organisation, Management and health delivery system in India.
2. **Hospital Pharmacy:**
   (a) Definition
   (b) Functions and Objectives of Hospital Pharmaceutical Services
   (c) Location, Layout, Flow Chart of Materials and Men
   (d) Personnel and facilities requirements including equipment based on individual and basic needs
   (e) Requirements and abilities required for Hospital Pharmacists.
3. **Drug Distribution system in Hospitals**
   (a) Out-patient services
   (b) In patient services: (i) Types of services (ii) Detailed discussion of Unit dose system, Floor ward stock system, Satellite pharmacy services, Central sterile services, Bed Side Pharmacy.
4. **Manufacturing**
   (a) Economical considerations, Estimation of demand.
   (b) Sterile manufacture - Large and small volume parenterals, Facilities, requirements, Layout, Production planning, Man-power requirements.
   (c) Non-sterile manufacture - Liquid orals, Externals, Bulk concentrates.
   (d) Procurement of stores and testing of raw materials.
5. Nomenclature and Uses of Surgical Instruments and Hospital Equipments and Health Accessories.
6. P.T.C. (Pharmacy) and Therapeutic Committee), Hospital Formulary System and their Organisation, Functioning, Composition.
7. Drug Information service and Drug Information Bulletin.
8. Surgical dressing like Cotton, Gauge, bandages and Adhesive tapes including their pharmacopoeial test for quality. Other hospital supply e.g. I.V. sets, B. G. sets, Ryals tubes, Catheters, Syringes, etc.
9. Application of computers in maintenance of records, inventory control, medication monitoring, drug information and data storage and retrieval in hospital and retail pharmacy establishments.

PART - II : CLINICAL PHARMACY

1. Introduction to Clinical Pharmacy Practice - Definition, Scope.
2. Modern Dispensing Aspects - Pharmacists and Patient Counselling and Advice for the use of common drugs, Medication history.
3. Common daily terminology used in the Practice of Medicine.
4. Disease, Manifestations and Pathophysiology including salient symptoms to understand the diseases like Tuberculosis, Hepatitis, Rheumatoid Arthritis, Cardio-Vascular diseases, Epilepsy, Diabetes, Peptic Ulcer, Hypertension.
5. Physiological Parameters with their Significance.
6. Drug Interactions.
   (a) Definition and Introduction.
   (b) Mechanism of Drug Interaction.
   (c) Drug-drug interaction with reference to analgesics, diuretics, cardiovascular drugs. Gastro-intestinal agent, Vitamins and Hypoglycemic agents.
   (d) Drug-food interaction.
7. Adverse Drug Reactions
   (a) Definition and Significance.
   (b) Drug - induced diseases and Teratogenicity.
8. Drugs in Clinical Toxicity - Introduction, General treatment of poisoning, Systematic antidotes. Treatment for insecticide poisoning heavy metal poison, Narcotic drugs, Barbiturate, Organophosphorus poisons.
9. Drug dependences, Drug abuse, Addictive drugs and their treatment complications.
10. Bio-availability of drugs, including factors affecting it.

***

Contents ...

PART - I : HOSPITAL PHARMACY

PART - II : HOSPITAL PHARMACY

***

Part I - Hospital Pharmacy

1

HOSPITAL

Definition

A hospital is an establishment where medical or surgical care and treatment is provided for the ill or injured by a team of trained staff using specialized scientific equipment. It provides a range of health care services which include medical, surgical, psychiatric, testing and diagnostic services and treatment. These services are co-ordinated within a hospital with the aim to restore and maintain good health.

It is a place where resources like (a) Services of health care professionals, (b) Physical facilities and specialized equipment and (c) Funds are organised, put together and utilized to fulfil the health care needs of a community. Thus a hospital is a complex organisation which works with an objective of restorating and improving the health status of a community at large. Hospitals in earlier days were charitable institutes which took care of the sick who were needy, aged or infirm. They were set up to basically look after the homeless sick.

Today modern hospitals are not just centres of cure but centres of promotion of health They provide 'medical care' which encompasses preventive, curative and even rehabilitative measures.

The growth and development of hospitals to expand to their modern day role is due to factors like

1. Realisation of importance of good health by the public at large.
2. Public awareness regarding preventive health care.
3. Advances in medical and related biological sciences.
4. Assuarance about the quality of care provided by the hospitals; creating faith in the minds of people.
5. Time demanded needs about health care like wounded soldiers in world wars or victims of Epidemics etc.

Functions of a Hospital

The main functions of a hospital are:

(i) Patient care.

(ii) Training of medical and health professionals and patients.

(iii) Medical Research.

(iv) Public health.

Patient Care: The main function of a hospital is to provide care to the sick or injured and restore the health of the patient. It raises the quality of care and general standards of medical practice. It is a centre of community health and contributes a great deal to preventive and social medicine,

Training of Medical and Health Professionals and Patient: Training or education is an important function of a hospital. Education in a hospital has two different forms namely, (i) educating the medical and health professionals and (ii) educating the patient. A hospital could be considered as a workshop where the student learns by observing and practicing under the supervision of his superiors. Training to the nurses, medical and social workers, X-ray and laboratory technicians and other staff is an essential facet of hospitals. Such trainings programmes should be arranged periodically under the supervision of experienced superiors. A hospital also aims to educate the general public through lectures and demonstrations on the preventive aspects of common and serious diseases. A hospital provides the means and methods by which persons can work together in groups to take care of patients and the community. Hospitals provide facilities for continuing education all persons involved in health care, patients and their relatives.

Medical Research

Hospital research is important as it helps in developing new methods of treatment and improving a hospital services. Some of the common areas of research in a hospital are development of new techniques in surgery, laboratory diagnostic procedures, evaluation of investigational drugs in diseases etc. It helps to lower incidences of disease through early detection and treatment. It also helps to develop and maintain an effective system of clinical and administrative records and reports. Hospitals also participate in the financial plan and safety programmes.

Public health: Hospitals are required to support all the activities carried out by various public health and voluntary agencies such as immunization programmes, blood donation camps, social and economic rehabilitation, health education etc. by providing facilities and advice.

Classification of Hospital

Hospitals are classified in different ways and a hospital could fall under more than one category. There are three basic classifications of hospital based on (i) the type of clinical services offered, (ii) the length of stay and (iii) the ownership/control of hospital.

1. Clinical Services Offered: Clinical services offered by hospitals are either specialized or general. Most Government hospitals usually offer general hospital services, providing a wide range of service areas such as surgical, internal medicine, orthopedic, dental and obstetric care. The specialized care include medicine and surgery.

Clinical services

- General
- Specialized
  - Medicine
    - (a) Tuberculosis
    - (b) Internal medicine
    - (c) Paediatrics
    - (d) Psychiatrics and nervous diseases
    - (e) Communicable diseases
  - Surgery
    - (a) Orthopedic
    - (b) Otolaryngologic
    - (c) Gynaecologic
    - (d) Ophthalmic

2. Length of stay:

(a) Short term (Acute): Average length of stay of patient is less than 30 days.

(b) Long term (Chronic): Length of stay of patient is more than 30 days.

e.g. Psychiatric condition.

3. Ownership and Control Basis: The group that controls, owns or operates the hospital may be either Governmental or voluntary organisations (Non-Governmental).

(a) Governmental: This includes those hospitals that are owned and/or operated by an agency of the central/state government, or other political subdivisions of Government.

Governmental

- **Central Government**
  e.g. 1. All India institute of medical sciences and hospital, Delhi
  2. Central Govt. health scheme hospitals
- **State Government**
  e.g. 1. Civil hospitals
  2. Cottage hospitals
  3. Primary health centres.
- **Others**
  e.g. 1. Military hospitals
  2. Corporation hospital

(b) Non-Governmental:

(i) Private: (a) Profit (b) Non-profit.

(ii) Community

Hospitals can also be classified on the basis of:

1. Accreditation: In the United States, hospitals are also classified on the basis of accreditation procedure which considers the compliance to specified standards of health care.

(a) Accredited

(b) Non-accredited.

2. **Teaching hospital:** A teaching hospital is one where clinical instruction is imparted to medical school students. Teaching hospitals are the places where new medical graduates undergo 1 year of hospital training and get experience in a broader perspective in clinical care of patients, teaching and research.

3. **Capacity:** The hospitals are also classified on the basis of bed capacity as :

Under 50 beds	200-299 beds
50-99 beds	300-399 beds
100-199 beds	400-499 beds
	500 and over beds

Clinic: A clinic is an establishment where ambulatory patients are admitted for special study and treatment by a group of physicians practicing together, and where the patient is not confined as in a hospital.

Hospital Organisation: The organisation and management of a hospital differs based on the type of hospital and on the ownership and control of hospital.

In the case of a smaller hospital there are fewer administrative positions of associate or assistant directors whereas in larger hospitals, the general areas of clinical and administrative services may be further subdivided in units. The corporation and the board of trustees segment of the organisation is standard for all private hospitals. Government hospitals usually have a board of trustees but no corporate body.

A representative organisational chart of a hospital is shown here:

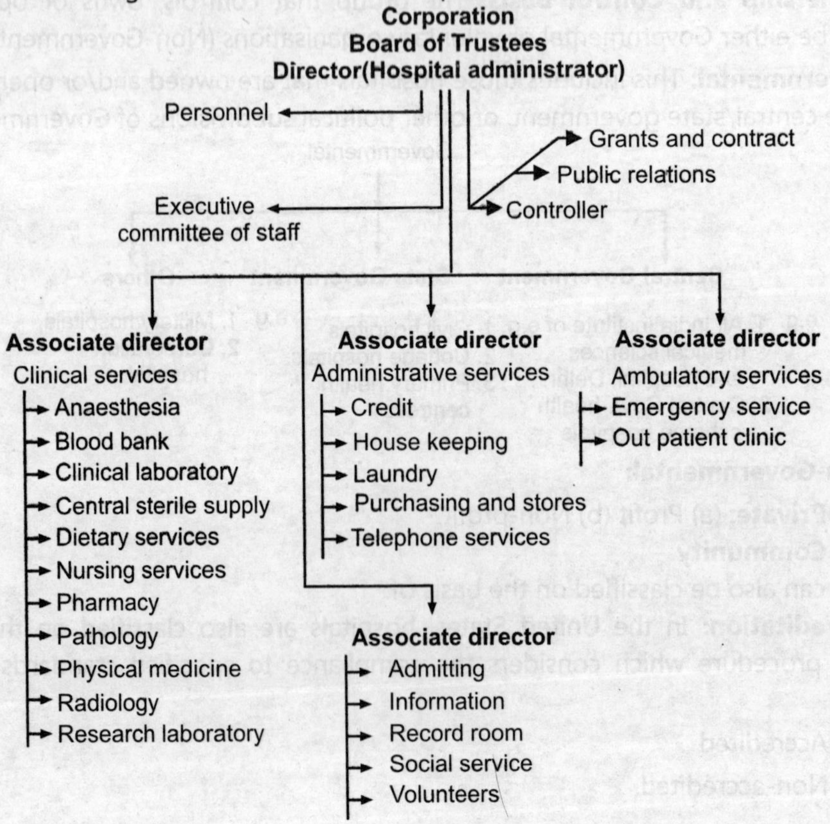

The organisational structure of a medical centre teaching hospital is shown in the chart below.

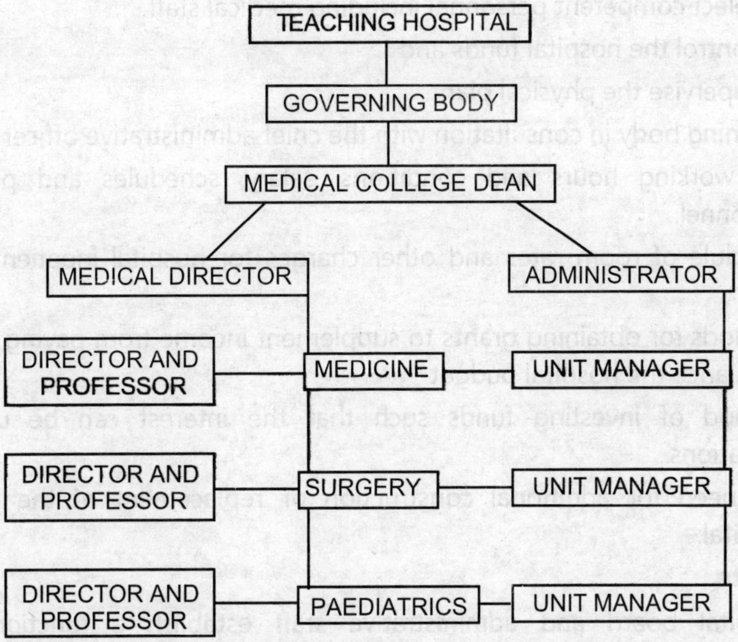

Governing Body and Management

Regardless of the kind of organisation and control a hospital is under, there is always some sort of a governing body to which the administrator must report.

In state, country and city hospitals the governing body is usually from some political subdivision, whereas in the non-profit, non-government hospital there is usually a governing board which takes the overall responsibility for the proper functioning of the hospital such that adequate service can be rendered to the patient at as low a cost as possible with maximum efficiency.

Most hospitals in the United States need not just a license but also require recognition by the Joint Commission on Accreditation on Hospitals (JCAH) as an accredited hospital. The purposes of JCAH are :

1. To establish the standards of the hospital.
2. To conduct surveys and accreditation programmes for following purposes:
   (a) To promote high quality care in all aspects.
   (b) To apply certain basic principles of physical plant safety and maintenance.
   (c) To maintain the essential services through the coordinated effort of the staff.
3. To recognise compliance of standards by issuing certificates of accreditation.
4. To conduct educational and research programmes and publish the results thereof.

Functions of the Governing Body

1. To select competent personnel including medical staff.
2. To control the hospital funds and
3. To supervise the physical plant.

The governing body in consultation with the chief administrative officer must establish:

(a) The working hours and conditions, salary, schedules and proper checks on personnel.

(b) Schedule of room rates and other charges for hospital inpatient and ambulatory care.

(c) Methods for obtaining grants to supplement income from paying patients and help to balance the hospital budget.

(d) Method of investing funds such that the interest can be used for hospital operations.

(e) The need for additional construction or replacement of the physical plant of hospital.

Departments

The hospital board and administrative staff establish a functional departmental organisation. The number and size of departments in any hospital orgaisation vary with the type and size of the hospital and with the area served (in terms of population and specific needs). Basically, these departments may be divided into general service, administration departments and clinical departments. The following chart shows hospital organisation and its administration and professional services in relation to the patient.

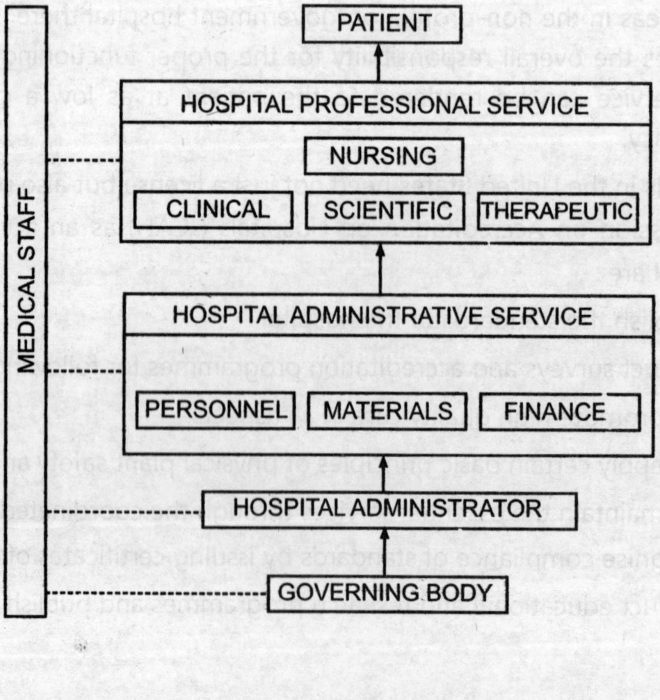

Medical Staff of the Hospital

The duties of the organised medical staff after its approval by the governing body are as follows:

(a) To provide professional care to sick and injured patients.

(b) To participate in the educational programme of the hospital.

(c) To audit their own professional work.

(d) To maintain their own efficiency.

(e) To advise and assist the administrator and governing body regarding medical policies.

The medical staff consists of the following groups :

1. Honorary staff
2. Consulting staff
3. Active staff
4. Associate staff
5. Courtesy staff
6. Resident staff

The honorary medical staff consists of physicians who are active in the hospital despite having retired. They continue to serve in the hospital because of their vast experience, indepth knowledge and outstanding work. This is a way of honouring them.

The consulting medical staff consists of specialists from various faculties, who are past speciality board members or belong to a national organisation.

The active or attending medical staff is the group most actively involved in the hospital. They are concerned with the care of all the patients in the hospital.

The associate medical staff is a group of junior or less experienced members.

Courtesy medical staff is a group of physicians who have the priviledge of attending to their own private patients at the hospital. They are not involved in the treatment of other patients in the hospital.

The resident medical staff is a group of physicians who are employees of the hospital residing in the campus.

The Supporting Services

The clinical department of the hospital would not be able to function without the following supporting services :

(a) Anaesthesia Service: Anaesthesia care is usually provided by anaesthesiologist or qualified physician anesthetist and qualified nurse anaesthetist. The anaesthesia service of hospital is generally directed by a physician member of the medical staff who has had a special training and is responsible for the following:

(i) quality of anaesthesia care.

(ii) availability of equipment required for administration of anaesthetic.

(iii) development of regulations and evaluation of anaesthesia care.

(b) Blood Bank: Most hospitals have a blood bank as blood is required frequently. The blood supply service is generally under the supervision of a licensed physician. In some hospitals, the blood supply service is assigned to the pathology department. Depending on the hospital size, an adequate supply of blood may be maintained in the hospital's own blood bank.

(c) Central Sterile Supply: This supplies all the necessary requirements in sterile condition to nursing units which include needles, syringes, linen and other surgical supplies.

(d) Dietary Services: A dietician is a qualified individual who has studied the science and principles of nutrition. A dietician applies the principles of nutrition effectively to the dietary service provided by the hospital.

The dietician is generally responsible for recording dietary histories of patients who have food allergies or restricted diets.

(e) Nursing Services: Nursing service is important in the hospital for the following reasons:

(i) It encompases health promotion, care and prevention of disease, rehabilitation, teaching, counselling and emotional support.

(ii) It is an integral part of total health care and is planner and administered in combination with related medical, educational and welfare services.

(iii) Nursing personnel respect individuality, dignity and rights of every person regardless of race, colour and social or economic status.

(f) Medical Records Service: Every hospital is required to maintain adequate medical records of their patients.

The following are the purposes of keeping the medical records:

1. It serves as a basis for planning and continuity of patient care.
2. It provides the means of communication among the physician and nursing staff.
3. It serves as a basis for study and evaluation of the care rendered to the patient.
4. It provides data for use in research education.
5. It furnishes documentary evidence for the course of patient's illness and treatment during each hospital stay.

The medical records must include all the detailed clinical information to enable another practitioner to give effective continuing care to patient and a consultant to give an opinion after his examination of the patient.

A complete medical record includes:

(i) Identification and sociological data.

(ii) Family history and present illness.

(iii) Physical examination data.

(iv) Special examination data: Clinical, laboratory data, X-ray findings.

(v) Provisional diagnosis.

(vi) Medical or surgical treatment.

(vii) Microscopic pathologic findings.

(viii) Progress notes.

(ix) Final diagnosis.

(x) Condition on discharge.

(xi) Autopsy findings.

(g) Pathology Services: These services analyse samples such as blood, urine, faeces, sputum, semen for the presence of microorganisms and abnormal constituents. The samples are analysed for their normal composition also. The head of the pathology laboratory is a member of the medical staff.

(h) Radiology: This department of the hospital is necessary for diagnostic and thereapeutic purposes. The department is under the supervision of a qualified physician who is trained and experienced in general radiology. These services are performed only on receipt of a written order by a member of the medical staff.

Hospital Management

The Management process of any business involves the following: Planning, Organising, Staffing, Directing, Controlling, Reviewing, Communicating, Co-ordinating and Decision-making.

Directing

1. On-duty and Work Schedules: Some departments such as 'nursing' need staff on duty every hour, every day and some such as 'catering' two shifts every day. Other departments such as Administration and business require staff on duty Monday to Friday with 'on-call' arrangements.

Work schedules are routine tasks listed in order of performance and the workers to whom they are assigned. Tasks are specific as to what is to be done, where and during what time?

2. Job Introduction: Helping new workers adjust to their job and work situation is called job introduction. It entails:

(a) Welcome by the department manager.

(b) Introduction to colleagues.

(c) Broad explanation of department work.

(d) Explanation of worker's own duties

(e) Administrative schedules.

(f) On-duty and work schedules.

Effective job introduction reduces a new worker's anxieties and it should be given by the department manager on the first day of employment.

3. Training: It helps workers to acquire and develop skills for effective and efficient work performance. It helps in:

(i) Reducing labour turnover.

(ii) Reducing health and injury hazard.

(iii) Giving a sense of job security.

(iv) Increasing promotion opportunities and raising morale.

(v) Facilitating exchange of jobs between workers.

Training is needed for new staff as well as for operating new equipment. Hospital training methods include 'on-the-job', apprenticeship and programmed instruction. Other training methods include discussions, conferences, seminars, workshops, demonstrations and lectures.

4. Supervision: It is the verbal or written direction to subordinates for commencing, modifying or stopping an activity. In a hospital, according to the necessity or emergency, supervisory directions are essential.

Controlling: It may be quantitative (e.g. the number of patients admitted) or qualitative (e.g. controlling the clarity of radiograph). The control on narcotics is stricter than aspirin tablets.

Information is needed on actual performance such as the number of patients, days of care provided, and resources used such as money. Controlling information includes statistics which measure actual performance in quantitative terms such as surgical operations performed and the number of operating room hours needed. The information obtained is evaluated by the departmental manager and corrective action if necessary is taken by the person in charge.

The corrective action may be prompt and vigorous adjustment of activities so that actual performance is consistent with expected performance. This action is facilitated by knowing location, time and worker, for deviations caused. The root cause of deviations should be sought e.g. late delivery of clean linen to the wards may be caused not by laundering delays but by transportation delays. Work schedules may need revising. Workers and supervisors may need more training. The corrective action may require raising of morale and increasing motivation of workers.

Health Delivery System in India

The central government has a "Union Ministry of Health and Family Welfare" and the state government has a "Ministry of Health" which formulates and plans the overall health policy and health schemes.

The following chart explains the organisation of health delivery system.

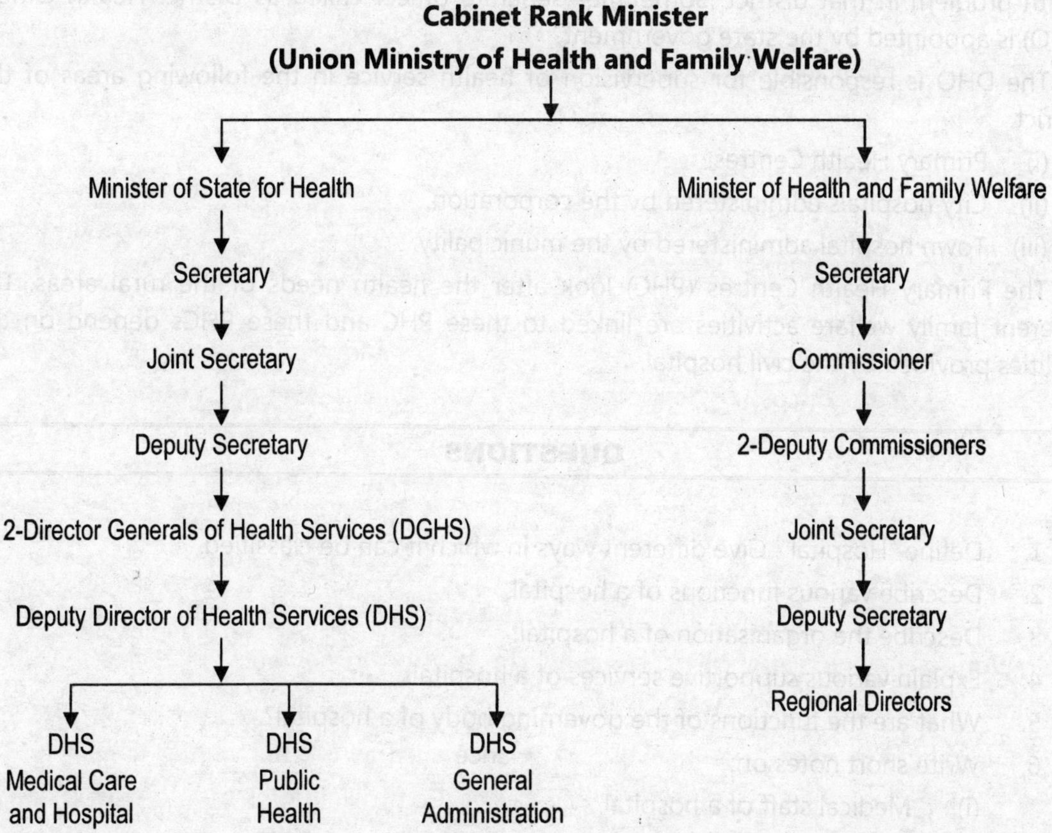

Organisational Structure of Health Delivery System at State Level

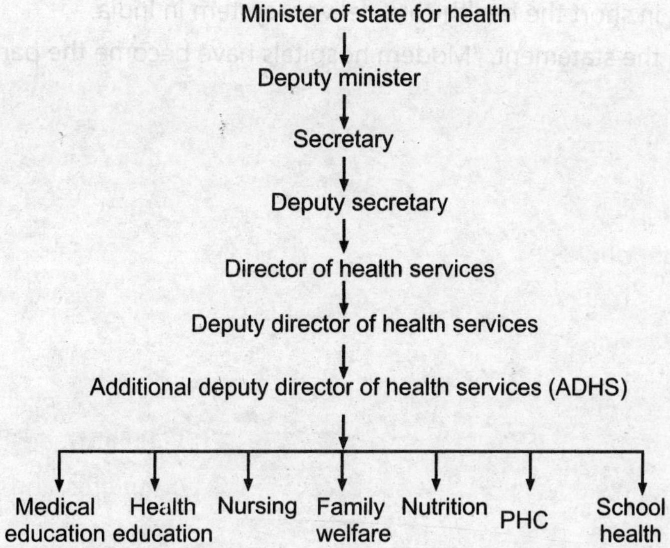

A Chief Medical Officer (CMO) is appointed for each district and is responsible for any health problem in that district. Sometimes separate officer called as District Health Officer (DHO) is appointed by the state government.

The DHO is responsible for supervision of health service in the following areas of the district.

(i) Primary Health Centres.

(ii) City hospitals administered by the corporation.

(iii) Town hospital administered by the municipality.

The Primary Health Centres (PHC) look after the health needs of the rural areas. The different family welfare activities are linked to these PHC and these PHCs depend on the facilities provided by the civil hospital.

QUESTIONS

1. Define "Hospital". Give different ways in which it can be classified.
2. Describe various functions of a hospital.
3. Describe the organisation of a hospital.
4. Explain various supportive services of a hospital.
5. What are the functions of the governing body of a hospital?
6. Write short notes on:
   (i) Medical staff of a hospital.
   (ii) Medical records services.
   (iii) Governing body and management.
   (iv) Nursing services.
7. Explain in short the health care delivery system in India.
8. Explain the statement, "Modem hospitals have become the part of our life."

***

2

HOSPITAL PHARMACY

In the past several decades, there have been considerable advances and developments in the field of pharmacy. Numerous drugs have been isolated and synthesized in the last few years which have lcd to advance in medical treatments. However many of these drugs had side effects which could complicate the existing health problem. Basically, a pharmacist is concerned with manufacture, quality control, research and development, storage, distribution and administration of the pharmaceutical products.

A hospital pharmacist was the first recognised representative of the pharmaceutical profession. The first North American Hospital, Pennsylvania Hospital started functioning in 1752 and Jonathan Roberts worked in it as a Hospital Pharmacist. The greatest achievements in the profession were made in early 1940s. The American Society of Hospital Pharmacists was formed in 1942 and they published the American journal of Hospital Pharmacy. In 1946, there were approximately 7000 hospitals registered by the American Hospital Association, however by 1977, the number increased to 7,099. With an increase in the number of hospitals, the purchase and use of drugs increased, which in turn necessitated the modernization of hospitals. The hospital administrator realized that only trained pharmaceutical personnel were capable of storing, handling, pricing and dispensing pharmaceutical products.

Hospital Pharmacy is defined as the actual practice of pharmacy in a hospital. This department in the hospital, under the supervision of professionally competent and legally qualified pharmacists and from where:

(a) All medications are supplied to the nursing units.

(b) Special prescriptions are filled for in-patients and outpatients.

(c) Pharmaceuticals are manufactured in bulk.

(d) Narcotics, biologicals and prescribed drugs are dispensed.

(e) Injectables are prepared and sterilised and

(f) Professional supplies are often stocked and dispensed.

Functions of Hospital Pharmacy

The hospital pharmacy is one of the many departments of the hospital and it has in general following basic functions:

1. To provide and evaluate service in support of medical care for achieving the objectives and policies of hospital.

2. To implement the philosophy, objectives, policies and standards of the hospital.
3. To participate in the functioning of all other department and services of the hospital.
4. To estimate the requirements of the department and to recommend and implement policies and procedures to maintain an adequate and competent staff.
5. To develop and maintain an effective system of clinical and/or administrative records and reports.
6. To estimate the requirements for facilities, supplies any equipments.
7. To co-ordinate with the financial plan of operation for the hospital.
8. To initiate and participate in studies or research project designed for the improvement of health care of patients and other hospital services.
9. To provide and implement continuing education in pharmacy programme for all health professionals in the hospital.
10. To initiate and participate in the safety programme of the hospital.

Objectives of Hospital Pharmacy

The objectives of hospital pharmacy are to draw the plans and implement them for the following purposes:

1. To teach the hospital pharmacist about the philosophy and ethics of hospital pharmacy and guide them to take responsibility for professional practice.
2. To strengthen the management skills of hospital pharmacist working as the head of the department.
3. To strengthen the scientific and professional aspects of practice of hospital pharmacy such as consulting role of hospital pharmacist, his teaching role and research activities.
4. To utilise as maximum as possible the resources of hospital pharmacy for the development of the profession.
5. To attract greater number of well trained pharmacists to work in the hospital pharmacy.
6. To promote the payment of good salaries to hospital pharmacist in order to retain the services of these professionals.

Location and Lay-out of Hospital Pharmacy

The location of a hospital pharmacy should be such that it is convenient for providing service to all departments of hospital and personnel who make daily use of such service.

In a general hospital of less than 200 beds, the pharmacy should be located on the first floor in the centre and near to the out-patient department (if present in hospital). This will increase the efficiency and reduce the man-hours of work.

In majority of hospitals, pharmacy serving in-patient and out-patient facility is constructed.

Floor-space Requirement

The recommended floor space requirement for general hospital pharmacies is given below:

Area in Sq. ft. for	50 Beds	100 Beds	200 Beds
1. Compounding and dispensing laboratory	205	320	495
2. Parenteral solutions laboratory		185	200
3. Store Room		125	200
4. Manufacturing laboratory			120
5. Office and Library			105
6. Circulation			60
Total	**205**	**630**	**1,180**

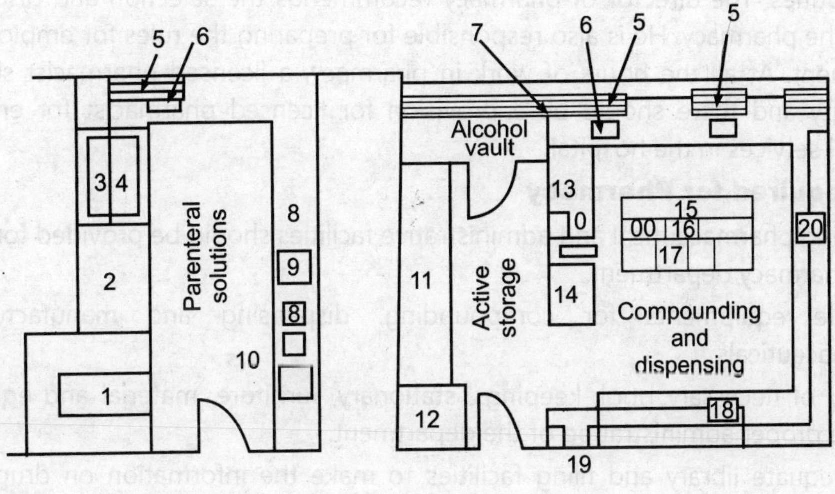

Corridor

(1) Sterilizer (2) Cabinet, storage, (3) Cabinet, adjustable shelves, (4) Sterilizer under counter, (5) Guards at all windows, (6) Hot plate, (7) Heat outlet grill, (8) Rack, bottle, (9) Tank, distilled water, (10) Sink, two compartments, (11) Shelves, (12) Dumbwaiter, (13) Desk: (a) Telephone outlet, (b) Waste papers, (14) Refrigerator, (15) Counter, (16) Rack, (17) Cabinets, (18) Scale prescription, (19) Window, dispensing, (20) Sink.

Fig. 2.1: Pharmacy Department for General Hospital of 100 Beds

Requirements for Personnel in a Hospital Pharmacy

The director of pharmacy should be a graduate of an accredited college of pharmacy or a Bachelor of science with at least one year experience in hospital pharmacy. He should have an adequate number of assistants who are licensed pharmacists to supply highest quality of pharmaceutical service.

Personnel required for Hospital Pharmacy are:

(a) Director of pharmacy.

(b) One or more assistant directors of pharmacy.

(c) Staff pharmacists.

(d) Residents.

(e) Personnel trained in non-professional function and clerical help.

The director of pharmacy service should have completed three years course but if he does not have B. S. degree he should have 5 years experience in hospital pharmacy and if the director have completed 2 years course in pharmacy but does not have B. S. degree he should have 10 years of experience in hospital pharmacy. The selection of the resident personnel would be on the basis of minimum standards established for the residency program. The selected personnel should be graduates and licensed pharmacists.

In order to give the best pharmaceutical services, the non-professionals should not be assigned any duties. The director of pharmacy recommends the selection and discharge of employees in the pharmacy. He is also responsible for preparing the rules for employees and their enforcement. At all the hours of work in pharmacy, a licensed pharmacist should be present on duty and there should be a provision for licensed pharmacist for emergency pharmaceutical services in the hospital.

Facilities Required for Pharmacy

The following pharmaceutical and administrative facilities should be provided for efficient running of a pharmacy department.

(a) Suitable equipments for compounding, dispensing and manufacturing of pharmaceuticals.

(b) Supply of necessary book-keepings, stationary, furniture, material and equipments for the proper administration of the department.

(c) An adequate library and filing facilities to make the information on drugs readily available to both physician and pharmacist. A modern pharmaceutical library should be maintained in which following official books and journals should be available:

- National Formulary,
- United States Pharmacopoeia,
- American Hospital Formulary Service,
- Journal of American Pharmaceutical Association,
- International Pharmaceutical Abstracts,
- Journal of Pharmaceutical Sciences,
- American Journal of Hospital Pharmacy and
- Journal of American Medical Association.

The library should contain the text and reference books on the following subjects.

Pharmacy, Chemistry, Pharmacology, Bacteriology, Toxicology, Therapeutics, Staining Techniques; Sterilization and Disinfection Techniques and Medical Dictionary.

The library should contain other publications on "Recent Advances in Pharmaceutical Services."

(d) Adequate locking arrangement for storage of narcotics, alcohol.

(e) Sufficient floor space with proper lighting and ventilation should be provided for adequate storage of pharmaceuticals and other operations of pharmacy.

(f) The facility of refrigerator should be provided for the storage of thermolabile products.

Equipments Required for Pharmacy

The list of equipments required for the pharmacy department should be prepared in consultation with other departments of the hospital. The equipments should be selected in such a way that these will provide good service with minimum maintenance cost within hospital's equipment budget.

The equipments required are of two types:

1. **Fixed equipments:** These are equipments which require installation and are fixed to the building. These are items which are included in construction contracts of the building e.g. cabinets, counters, dumbwaiters, elevators and sinks.

2. **Movable equipments:** These are equipments which can be moved and which are not meant to be permanently fixed to the building. These are large number of items of furniture and equipments having reasonably fixed position but can be moved. e.g. Balances, desks, mixers, carts etc.

Since, the services rendered by each hospital pharmacy vary from hospital to hospital, it is difficult to prepare a standard list of equipments. The United States Public Health Service has suggested an equipment list according to bed capacity.

(A) For Inpatient Dispensing	**Suggested Quantity for Number of Beds**		
Fixed equipments	**100**	**300**	**500**
1. Cabinets (Wall mounted)			
2. Counter prescription	1	3	6
3. Dumbwaiter	1	1	1
4. Pneumatic tube station	0	1	1
5. Shelf adjustable 12"	1	2	3
6. Ledge fixed	0	1	1
Movable Equipments			
1. Cabinet, filing, 5-drawer	1	1	0
2. Cart, delivery, large	0	1	2
3. Refrigerator			
(a) Biological type with freezer	1	0	0
(b) Pass-through, cafeteria type for IV solutions	0	1	1
(c) Open front, refrigerated case type	0	1	1
4. Type writers, electric, non-movable carriage	1	2	4
5. Stool, operators, adjustable	1	2	4

(B) For Out-patient Dispensing			
1. Cabinet, wall-mounted	–	1	–
2. Counter with sink, drainboard, file drawer	–	1	
3. Counter with file drawer, bins and shelf	1	1	
4. Door, flexible, pull down type for outpatient dispensing counter window	1	1	–
5. Panels, acoustial	–	1	–
6. Shelving, adjustable, wall mounted 12"	1		
Movable Equipments			
1. Cabinet, filing, rotary, mechanical	–	1	–
2. Chairs for waiting area	–	4	–
3. File, Swinging panel, strip insert	1	1	
4. Refrigerator, Biological with freezer	–	1	
5. Waste receptacle	1	–	

Responsibilities of Hospital Pharmacist

The responsibilities are given below departmentwise:

(A) Inpatient Pharmacy Department

(I) Dispensing area:

1. **Policies:** He ensures that the established policies and procedures of the hospital are followed.
2. **Accuracy:** He keeps the proper control for the accuracy of dosages prepared especially for intravenous administration.
3. **Maintenance of records:** He keeps the records of drugs supplied, drugs returned, bills of investigational drugs and I.V. admixtures, etc.
4. **Storage:** He keeps an adequate control over the drugs stored in his section.
5. **Working:** He ensures that all laws and rules are followed in his section and adequate techniques are used for compounding the preparations.
6. **Co-ordination:** He co-ordinates all the activities of the dispensing area to give the best possible service.
7. **Drug Information:** He keeps himself and his staff well informed about the drugs stored in the hospital, about their side effects, therapeutic efficacy and stability etc.

(II) Patient Care Area:

1. **Co-ordination:** He co-ordinates all the pharmacy services in the nursing unit.
2. **Communication:** He communicates with nurses and medical staff regarding medication administration problems.

3. **Technical:** (a) He gives instructions to the technicians regarding the new procedures and dealing with difficult patients. (b) He acts as a link between the technician and nursing and medical staff and ensures that proper techniques are used by the technician for administering the drugs. (c) He assists in training new technicians. (d) He ensures that adequate number of technicians are provided to inpatient care area. He ensures that technicians are following the personnel policies and rules and keeping the medication area neat.
4. **Supervisory:** (a) He reviews all medication orders to ensure that these are entered accurately in the unit dose system. (b) He periodically inspects each patient's drug administration form to ensure that all doses are being administered and charted correctly. (c) He confirms periodically that administered doses are correctly noted on patient's chart and the drug charges are correctly assessed. (d) He reviews all doses missed, re-schedules the doses as necessary and signs all "Drugs not given" notices. (e) He periodically inspects the medication areas to ensure that adequate level of floor stock drugs and supplies are maintained.

(III) Direct Patient Care:

1. He obtains patient's medication history and gives the information to the physician.
2. He identifies the drugs brought in the hospital by patient.
3. **Patient monitoring:** The complete drug therapy of the patient for its effectiveness, side effects, toxicities, allergic reactions is monitored.
4. **Patient Counselling:** He helps in counselling the patient about self-administered drugs and discharge drugs.
5. **Selection of drug:** He assists the physician in selection of drug, dose regimens and schedules and the time for drug administration.
6. He participates in cardiopulmonary emergencies.

(IV) General Responsibilities:

He provides in-service education and drug information to all health professionals.

(B) Outpatient Pharmacist's Responsibilities:

(I) In dispensing area:

1. **Maintenance of records:** He provides for the adequate record keeping of the following: (a) Prescription files, (b) Outpatient bills, (c) Patient medication, (d) Investigational drugs, (e) Report.
2. **Co-ordination:** He co-ordinates all the activities of area with available staff to give the best possible service.
3. He ensures that proper personnels are present in the area with the proper knowledge of techniques and procedures to be followed.
4. He maintains the outpatients area neatly at all the times.
5. He maintains professional competence.

(II) Inpatient care area:

1. **Inspection:** He periodically inspects the medication area of the nursing unit for the proper supply and storage of stock drugs.
2. Patient monitoring and patient counselling as explained earlier.
3. In selection of drug therapy, dose regimen and schedule, he helps the physician and nursing staff.
4. He obtains patient's medication history and identifies drugs brought by him to the hospital and informs the same to the medical and nursing staff.

(III) General Responsibilities:

1. **Co-ordination:** He co-ordinates all the activities essential for providing the good ambulatory patient care.
2. **Drug Information:** He gives the adequate and essential drug information to all the health professionals.
3. **Control:** He provides good control over the proper handling of drugs and proper follow up of rules and procedures of the hospital.
4. **Education:** He provides in-service education and training programmes to all health professionals.
5. He maintains the professional competence in the area.
6. He participates in the cardio-pulmonary emergencies.

Qualifications of a Hospital Pharmacist

The pharmaceutical service of a hospital should be directed by a professionally competent and legally qualified pharmacist. Depending on the size and scope of the pharmaceutical services of the hospital, sufficient number of competent personnel should be available in the staff.

The director of the pharmaceutical services of the hospital should either be a graduate or post graduate from the college of pharmacy recognised by P.C.I. or should have completed hospital pharmacy training program. Consideration should be given to graduates of foreign colleges of pharmacy who are appropriately licensed. The preference should be given to personnel with Ph. D. (Pharmaceutical sciences) degree.

Abilities Required of Hospital Pharmacists

The American Society of Hospital Pharmacists and the American Association of colleges of pharmacy have developed and approved a statement on the Abilities Required of Hospital Pharmacists which is given below. A well qualified hospital pharmacist must possess the following abilities.

1. Administrative and Managerial Ability

The main administrative and managerial responsibilities of a hospital pharmacist include planning and integrating pharmacy policies, budgeting, stock control, maintenance of records and preparation of reports. He must be thoroughly familiar with the organisation of hospital, staff and line relationships and appropriate lines of communication. He co-ordinates the pharmacy activities with medical, nursing and other services of the hospital. He must be able to prepare suitable written communications to the hospital staff. He is responsible for interviewing and selecting the personnel for work in pharmacy. He organizes and schedules the work of pharmacy personnel. He is responsible for training and development of pharmacy personnel. He is responsible for justification and expenditure of pharmacy funds and keeping the records of all pharmacy operations.

2. Manufacturing Ability

Since a large number of hospitalized patients are served from the hospital pharmacy, he must be able to develop and conduct a pharmaceutical manufacturing program. He must be able to provide the drugs at a relatively low cost by manufacturing in bulk quantities. For this purpose he should have sufficient knowledge of availability and sources of drugs. He must be able to prepare and supply a required form of drugs which may not be commercially available.

3. Perfect Knowledge of

(a) Drugs and its actions: Since the hospital pharmacist and medical and nursing staff of the hospital are closely associated, he must have a perfect knowledge of drugs regarding its chemistry, pharmacology, toxic effects, routes of administration and other information. He also helps physicians in training by providing the information on drugs. He must be able to provide information on proper storage and handling of drugs. He must be able to apply his knowledge of drugs for individual cases of physicians and for dispensing a particular pharmaceutical quality of a drug.

(b) Control of drugs: In the hospital, he must be able to control not just the quality of drugs but also the distribution of drugs throughout the hospital.

- **(i) Quality control of drugs:** He must be able to develop and write specifications for drugs to be purchased and dispensed by the hospital pharmacy. For this purpose he must have the perfect knowledge of pharmaceutical properties of drugs. He must be able to evaluate the controls properly for selecting the manufactured drugs.
- **(ii) Control on distribution of drugs:** Depending on the type and size of hospital, the problem of drug distribution varies from hospital to hospital. This is important in case of patients requiring intensive drug therapy. Hence in large hospitals "automated" dispensing at nursing station is carried out.

4. Research Ability

Since the hospital pharmacist is the only person to identify the drugs being used, he helps in medical research to maintain the information of chemistry, pharmacology, toxicology, posology of compounds under investigation.

He must be able to perform pharmaceutical research on the drugs:

(a) To improve its usefulness.

(b) To develop methods for preservation and stability.

(c) To improve therapeutic effectiveness and taste.

(d) To develop the various bases and vehicles for improving the absorption of active ingredients from internal and external preparations.

5. Teaching Ability

He must be able to deliver lectures and give demonstrations for the nursing staff on:

(i) Methods of storage of drugs.

(ii) Drug usage.

(iii) Various dosage forms.

(iv) Mathematical calculations involving percentage solutions and dose calculation.

(v) Prescription writing.

(vi) Drug stability and incompatibilities.

He must be able to carry on a continuous training program for trainee and staff pharmacists.

It must be understood that no one person may possess all of the abilities cited above. Certainly a teaching or research hospital of large size provides more opportunity for the training programs and prepares the personnel skilled in any one of the areas or faculty.

QUESTIONS

1. Define "Hospital Pharmacy". Give the objective of hospital pharmacy.
2. What are the various functions of hospital pharmacy ?
3. Describe the requirements of personnel for pharmacy.
4. What are the different pharmaceutical and administrative facilities required for efficient running of pharmacy department ?
5. Write a note on "Equipments for pharmacy."
6. Describe the responsibilities of hospital pharmacist for
   (i) Inpatient pharmacy department.
   (ii) Outpatient pharmacy department.
7. Describe the qualifications and abilities required of hospital pharmacist.
8. Write short notes on:
   (i) Teaching and Research ability of hospital pharmacist.
   (ii) General responsibilities of an outpatient phamacist.

***

3

DRUG DISTRIBUTION SYSTEM IN HOSPITALS

A well planned and systematically laid out drug distribution system is extremely important in a hospital as it eliminates errors which could occur during the dispensing of drugs. This would then reduces the chances of drug interactions.

The system is categorized into two parts:

(i) Outpatient (outdoor) or Ambulatory patient.

(ii) Inpatient (Indoor).

Outpatients are those patients who are not admitted in the hospital. Outpatient dispensing is one of the basic functions of the pharmacy department in the hospital. The outpatient services of the hospital are classified into three categories.

(i) Primary care: This forms the major bulk of out patients. It includes a variety of services essential for maintaining the daily personal health.

(ii) Referral or tertiary care: It means the care of the patient beyond the primary care.

(iii) Emergency care: It is the care given to the patients suffering from serious health problems or accidents.

The following are the reasons for the development of outpatient department (O.P.D.) as a separate function of the hospital:

1. The demand by the community.
2. The need of the hospital and physician to have a greater control on patients receiving investigational use drugs.
3. The lack of sufficient number of physicians in some areas.
4. The need of the hospital to support its inpatient teaching programme.
5. The hospitals more active role in the community health programme.

The main advantages of dispensing medicines to outpatients are:

1. Treatment commences immediately.
2. Medicines may be prescribed as a part of clinical trial.
3. Medicines prescribed may be restricted to the hospital service.

Location or Outpatient Dispensing Service

There is no specific rule for location of outpatient dispensing service in a hospital. For location of this service three provisions are made:

(i) A separate outpatient dispensing pharmacy.

(ii) A combined unit service for in-patients and out-patients from same window and

(iii) A combined unit service for inpatients and outpatients from different windows.

However, the outpatient department and the pharmacy are geographically widely separated, a separate outpatient dispensing pharmacy needs to be set up. This arrangement has the advantage of a separate unit with a specialised function but possesses the disadvantages such as:

(i) It requires separate staff and

(ii) It is time consuming.

By using the combined unit service the above disadvantages are eliminated as well as the advantage is that the director of the pharmacy service is able to achieve a great degree of control and supervision.

Layout of Outpatient Service

The layout of this unit is important since it creates a good or bad impression about the hospital, depending on the services the outpatients get. The unit should be provided with two windows, one for receiving the prescription and other for delivery. A waiting area should be provided as the patients have to wait for same time while the prescription is being compounded. The waiting room should be clean and ventilated with sufficient number of comfortable seats. In the waiting room, general publications regarding pharmacy and medicines should be provided. It should also include magazines and news papers. The waiting period shouid be kept minimum to avoid overcrowding. In the waiting room the wall posters should be displayed through which the patients can learn about the family planning methods and general hygiene. The waiting room of outpatient dispensing unit could thus be utilised for educating the patients on matters relating to health and hygiene.

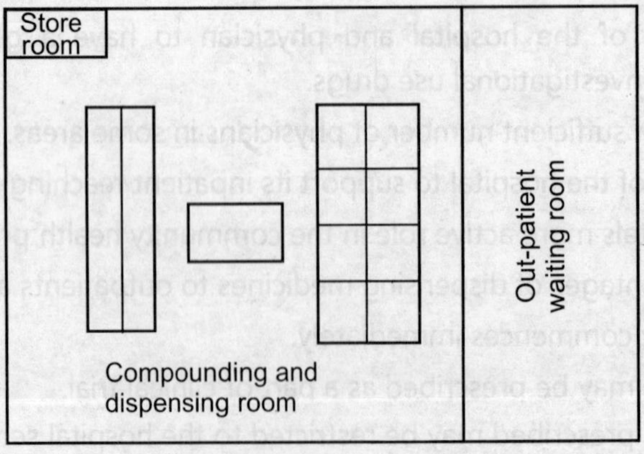

Fig. 3.1: A typical Out-patient Pharmacy. (Total area = 700 sq. ft.)

Dispensing Routine

Whenever the outpatient visits for the first time he should register his name at the registration office. Then he will be directed to a particular department where the physician would examine, diagnose the disease and writes the prescription. The prescription would bear the name, age, registration number and diagnosis of the patient. This prescription needs to be produced at the prescription receiving counter where the pharmacist checks the prescription and assembles the materials required for compounding. Most of the prescriptions are of the type pour and count the tablets or capsules.

The compounded prescription should be filled in a container and labelled. The label should indicate patient's name, registration number, age, and directions for use and storage.

The pharmacist should maintain a register for the purpose of accounting. He should retain the slips issued by the physician for tablets and capsules. The prescription needs usually given back to the patient so that the same can be produced by him during his next visit.

Drug Distribution System for Inpatients

An Inpatient is one who is confined to a bed or who is occupying a bed in the hospital.

Objectives: The objectives of drug distribution system for inpatients are:

(i) To provide drugs for all inpatients of the hospital on a 24 hours per day basis.

(ii) To inspect and control the distribution of drugs in all treatment areas.

Location, Layout and Planning

The unit should be located at such a place in the hospital which is readily accessible to all departments and free from disturbances.

The various sections of the inpatient pharmacy should be continuous. The unit should be well equipped. Operation of the satellite pharmacies should be supervised by a qualified pharmacist. The physical plan of this department should be well planned by considering the future growth of the hospital and to avoid the further modifications. The facilities and equipments used to store the drugs should be designed in such a way that it facilitates the routine inspection of the drugs before its administration and these are readily available to the physician and pharmacist.

Personnel for Inpatient Services

There is no standard rule for the requirement of personnel. It depends on the nature and quantum of service to be provided.

Hospital bed Strength	Number of Pharmacists
Upto 50	3
100	5
200	8
300	10
500	15

All these pharmacists should possess an adequate qualification in pharmacy and experience. If the pharmacy is also involved in the manufacture of drugs, then an adequate number of personnel need to be employed as pharmacy technicians, assistants, orderlies etc.

Methods of Drug Distribution

In hospital four drug distribution systems are used to distribute drugs from pharmacy to the wards:

(i) Individual prescription order system.

(ii) Floor stock system.

(iii) Combination of above two methods and

(iv) Unit dose dispensing.

(i) Individual Prescription Order System

All the medicines required for regular treatment are dispensed in the pharmacy department either by or under the direct supervision of a pharmacist, labelled with individual patient's name and instructions of dosage. The prescription sheets are usually sent to the pharmacy. This system is used only in small and private hospitals.

Advantages

1. Reduces manpower requirement.
2. All prescriptions are directly reviewed by the pharmacist.
3. Opportunity of close interaction between the pharmacist, nurse and physician.
4. It provides close control on stock.
5. Medication errors can be spotted.
6. Facilitates charging of private patients.

Disadvantages

1. Possibility of delay in obtaining medication.
2. Increases in the cost of drugs to patient.
3. It cannot be practised in big hospitals.

(ii) Complete Floor Stock System

Drugs are kept at the nursing stations. The drugs on the nursing station are of two types:

(a) Charge floor stock drugs: These are drugs which are stocked on the nursing station at all times and are charged to the patient's account after their administration to the patient.

(b) Non-charge floor stock drugs: These are drugs which are placed at the nursing station for the use of all patients in the ward and for which there may not be direct charge to patient's account. The cost of this group of drugs is calculated in the per day cost of hospital room.

Dispensing of charge floor stock drugs: The patients are charged mostly because of the high cost of drugs. These include injections or other single dose preparations. An envelope is used to dispense the drugs to the nursing station which is used as a charge ticket. The pre-labelled envelopes are filled with specific drugs in specified quantity and placed at the disposal of the nursing unit. When the drug is administered, the patient's name and room number is entered on the envelope and sent to the pharmacy.

Dispensing of Non-charge floor stock drugs

Two methods are used for the dispensing of non-charge or free floor stock drugs:

1. Drug Basket Method: The night nurse checks the medicine closet, utility room, and drugs supplies against a master list provided by the pharmacy. The nurse places a check mark on the number required for each drug on the requisition for floor stock supplies. She also places the empty containers in the drug basket. After completing the procedure, the empty containers and requisition for floor stock supplies is sent to the pharmacy. The pharmacy staff fills each container and dispenses the requested ampules and vials as ordered. Once the basket is completed, it is delivered to the floor.

2. Mobile Dispensing Unit: It is a specially constructed stainless steel body of the dimensions

Height - 60 inches

Width - 48 inches and

Depth - 25 inches

The body is fitted on six 8-inch balloon tyres, four of which are swivel type. The pharmacist controlling the mobile unit checks the items and quantity of supplies left in the pavilion drug cabinets. The carbon copy of the requisition for floor stock supplies is left on the pavilion as a record of the delivery and the original is returned to the pharmacy for the following purposes:

(i) To determine the rate of consumption of drugs.

(ii) To restock the mobile unit.

(iii) To serve as a charge document for the internal allocation of costs.

Advantages

1. The deteriorated, out-dated and non-approved drugs and drug samples may be removed quickly through the routine checking of the medicine cabinets. Thus, it eliminates drug returns.
2. The nursing station drug cabinets are under the continuous supervision of the pharmacist.
3. The pharmacist is available for spot consultation by the clinical and nursing staff.
4. Ready availability of required drugs.
5. Reduces pharmacy personnel.

Disadvantages

1. It consumes pharmacy personnel's time and

2. The inventory of the pavilion drug cabinets has to be done by the pharmacist and he has to check off the items and quantity of supplies left as the nurse will not do the same.

Selection of Charge Floor Stock Drugs

Pharmacy and therapeutic committee decides about the selection of drugs to be kept in the charge floor-stock. After fixing the floor stock, it is the responsibility of the hospital pharmacist to make the drugs available and also to re-submit the list of drugs for re-evaluation of newer needs to the committee.

The following types of drugs are usually stocked in the hospital:

Injectables

1. Antibiotics
   (a) Penicillin G Potassium 20 million units.
   (b) Procaine penicillin 300,000 units/ml.
   (c) Streptomycin sulphate 1 mg/2 ml.
2. Anti-epileptic
   Diphenyl hydantoin sodium - 50 mg/ml.
3. Antihypertensive
   Reserpine HCl 0.5 mg/2 ml.
4. Anticoagulant
   Heparin - 10,000 units/ml.
5. Coagulants
   Protamine sulphate 50 mg/5 ml.
6. Cardiovascular Agents
   (i) Depressant - Procainamide 100 mg/ml.
   (ii) Antifibrillator - Quinidine HCl 0.18/1.5 ml.
   (iii) Vasoconstrictor - Phenylephrine HCl 10 mg/ml.
   L - Arterenol 0-2%
   Metarenol Bitartarate 10 mg/ml.
7. Diuretics: Meralluride 2 ml
8. Anti-allergics
   Diphenylhydramine HCl 10 mg/ml.
   Hydrocortisone sodium succinate 100 mg.
9. Antinauseants
   Trimethobenzamide HCl 100 mg/ml.
   Prochlorperazine 10 mg/2 ml.
10. Spasmogenics
   Bethanecol chloride 5 mg/5 ml.

11. Tranquilizers
    Chlordiazepoxide 100 mg/ 2 ml.
12. Miscellaneous
    Polotassium chloride 49 mg/20 ml.
    Mannitol Injection 25%
    Dextrose 50%.

Selection of Non-charge Floor Stock Drugs

The selection of drug depends on:

1. Quantity of drug to be used.
2. The frequency of use.
3. The cost of the drug.
4. The effect on the hospital budget.

The list of drugs should be prepared by considering the need of the staff and the type of patients.

These are unit dose drugs and the cost is higher. Hence if there are frequent charges of the drug, the total charge of the drug may exceed the charge if it had been purchased in a multidose container. This could lead to bad public relations.

Labelling and Inspection of Floor Stock Drugs

Drugs are not labelled with directions for use in the ward stock. Both charge and non-charge floor stock drugs bear a label which indicates name of the ward, name and strength of the preparation and in case of some drug, the patient's name (for specific use only).

Because of large supply of drugs to the floor stock (nursing station), it is the responsibility of hospital pharmacist to inspect it regularly and to give the service adequately. The following points should be considered while inspecting the nursing drug cabinets:

1. Uniformity of containers.
2. Uniformity and completeness of labelling.
3. Whether lighting and refrigeration is functioning properly.
4. Various locks for security purpose.
5. No mixing of external and internal use products.
6. Check that drugs with date are still usable and whether the non-dated drugs have deteriorated.
7. Remove the samples, non-approved drugs or non-drug items from the nursing cabinet.
8. Check whether the research drugs are properly labelled.

Disadvantages of Complete Floor Stock System

1. Increased medication errors.
2. Greater pilferage, which increases during inventory.
3. Hazards due to improper storage facilities.
4. Increased nursing time on medication activity.
5. Nursing care is reduced.

(iii) Combination of Individual Prescription System and Floor Stock System

In this system drugs which are in frequent use are supplied as ward stocks and other drugs are individually dispensed when required.

(iv) Unit Dose Dispensing System

Unit dose medications can be defined as those medicines which are ordered, packaged, handled, administered and charged in multiples of single dose unit containing a predetermined amount of drug sufficient for one regular dose or application or use.

Advantages

1. The patients are charged only for those which are administered to them.
2. It reduces the medication error since the pharmacist checks a copy of physicians original order.
3. It avoids the drug losses.
4. Less space is required as compared to bulky floor stock.
5. Since all doses are prepared by the pharmacy it allows the nurses more time for direct patient care.
6. Patients receives the nursing service 24 hours a day.
7. It avoids duplication of orders and extra paper work.
8. It enhances more efficient utilization of personnel.

This system can be utilized in two ways:

1. Centralised unit dose drug distribution system and
2. Decentralised unit dose drug distribution system.

Centralised Unit Dose Dispensing

All drugs are stored in the central area pharmacy and dispensed at the time when it is required by the patient. This system can be used effectively by the use of medication carts and dumbwaiters for delivering the unit doses directly to the patient and for sending copies of physician's original medication order to pharmacy.

Decentralised Unit Dose Dispensing

This system consists of small satellite pharmacies located on each floor of the hospital. The centres such as storage, manufacturing, packaging which serves the satellites become the main pharmacy of this system. Medication carts are used for the delivery of drugs. Hospital with separate buildings uses this type of drug distribution system.

Procedure: After admitting patient in hospital, the data is filled on the patient profile card. The copies of the medication orders are sent to the pharmacist. The medication orders are entered on the patient profile card. The pharmacist checks the medication order for allergies, drug interactions and dosage schedule in consultation with nursing station. The medication cart is filled by the pharmacy technician according to dosage schedule delivery and is checked by the pharmacist before its release. The nurse administers the medication and makes the entry on her medication record. The cart is rechecked after returning to pharmacy. The pharmacist is available for consultation by doctors and nurses throughout the entire service.

Satellite Pharmacy Services

In a hospital where the main sections of pharmacy such as storing, manufacturing, dispensing are separated from each other, it is advisable to develop satellite pharmacies at the nursing station. In fact these are sub-pharmacies which receive their supplies from main pharmacy.

Advantages

1. Satellite pharmacies satisfactorily provide the required medication for a patient's current clinical needs.
2. The pharmacist of satellite pharmacy is available to patients and nursing professionals not just as a dispenser, but for clinical purposes also.
3. The pharmacist is present at the nursing station to perform the following:
   (a) Dispense unit doses and intravenous products.
   (b) Maintain patient drug policies.
   (c) Take patient drug histories.
   (d) Monitor patient for drug reactions and toxicity.

Central Sterile Services

A Central Sterile Supply Department (CSSD) in the hospital is one which receives used goods, processes to make them sterile and distributes and controls the sterile supplies to all units of hospital for the care and safety of the patient.

This department processes different surgical instruments, syringes, linen gloves, rubber and plastic goods, consumable dressing and suturing materials by using different methods of sterilization such as moist heat under pressure, dry heat, ethylene oxide and gamma radiations.

Location: It should be centrally located in the hospital or near a place where bulk of the supplies are required e.g. operation theatres which contributes about 75% of the work of this department. The stores and laundry should also be close by.

Layout of Central Sterile Service Department

While considering the layout of this department, care should be taken to segregate powder and fibre producing sections such as glove, dressing material and linen, as the presence of these into infusion or transfusion sets are hazardous to patient. Heat producing equipments such as distilled water still, storage tanks with heater, sterilizers etc. must be kept together and separated from the working place to provide comfortable working conditions for workers. It is essential to avoid mixing of clean things with dirty (unclean) things and sterile with non-sterile ones. This can be achieved by separating sterile and non-sterile area by centrally locating a battery of double door recessed type sterilizers with an emergency communication through air locks. Separate entrances are provided for both the areas. The glove room is at one corner end and dressing material section should be outside the main working area to reduce nuisance of powder and fibres in the area. The efficient working of any department depends upon the facilities provided in the form of adequate space, proper equipment and trained staff.

Space: The requirement of the space depends upon the services undertaken, the volume of work, degree of mechanisation, space for furniture, machines etc.

Staff: The department works for 24 hours to provide supplies. The staff appointed should be routinely sent for medical checkups and only medically fit staff should be kept in the department. Every member of the staff has to work with team spirit and contribute their knowledge and skill towards care and safety of the patient. The staff should maintain the required degree of cleanliness in daily work to minimise the bacterial count. The working according to the written procedures is essential to minimise errors and trouble to nursing staff, surgeons and finally to patients. The sterilised material should be handled carefully to avoid reinfection. Used material should be properly disinfected to avoid cross infections to worker as well as patient. To have a better service from the department following is essential:

1. Strict supervision over the working staff.
2. Proper control over quality, processing, storage and use.
3. Elimination of wastage of materials and staff working hours.
4. Maintenance of machines in working condition.
5. Introduction of production control, budgetory control and inventory controls.

By considering the above, it is possible to achieve the objective of proper care and safety of the patient.

Bed Side Pharmacy Services

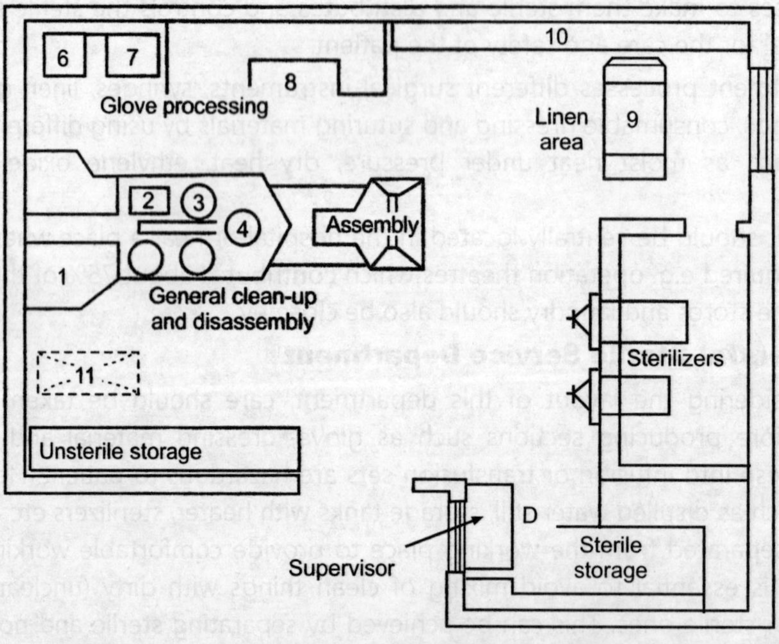

Fig. 3.2: Layout of Central Sterile Service Department

(1) General clean-up area (2) and
(3) Washing and rinsing area (4) Still
(5) Assembly station (6) and
(7) Glove washing, drying and powdering area (8) Glove packaging area
(9) Linen inspection and folding (10) Linen storage (11) CSR truck

As per the need for patient and if ordered by the doctor, 10 tablets of nitroglycerine are kept at the bed side. The nurse should count the number of tablets daily in the morning and evening and add the tablets (if used by the patient) to maintain the supply of ten tablets.

No medication except nitroglycerine is kept at the bed side of any patient. Medication brought to the hospital by patient is shown to the physician and then sent home with a responsible family member or friend.

Qualifications and Duties of Hospital Pharmacist to Manage Central Sterile Services

Since, the pharmacy students are exposed to the principles of sterilization, bacteriology, accounting and management, the hospital pharmacist is better qualified to manage central sterile services than a nurse. The pharmacist also has a better knowledge of use of products dispensed. Experience is also required for efficient operation.

The duties of hospital pharmacist in the area of central sterile services are:

1. Dispensing of supplies in small lots.
2. Purchasing of supplies.
3. Distribution of supplies towards various departments.
4. Discussions with sales personnel.
5. Arranging the meetings for discussion of procedures and problems concerning the services with medical staff.
6. Delivering the seminars and arranging the training programmes for various groups of personnel.
7. Manufacturing the various dosage forms in the hospital in small lots.
8. Practising the principle of standardisation.

This indicates that the pharmacist should be qualified both by education and experience to supervise the activities of central sterile supply services.

Standardization Committee

It is a group of persons within the hospital who are responsible for investigation, development and standardization of procedures and equipments. This group is also known as "Current Practices Committee". If such committee does not in exist in the hospital, then the director of pharmacy and central sterile supply services should take initial steps to form the committee that helps to reduce duplication of inventory and produces standardization of procedures.

The members of this committee should be appointed by the chief of the staff and the administrator of hospital from the following major areas of the hospital.

Administration (1)

Director of Laboratories:

Surgery (2)

Medicine (2)

Pathology (1)

Radiology (1)

Nursing service (2)

Nursing school (1)

Director of Pharmacy and Central Sterile Supply

Personnel should be invited from other areas of the hospital for meetings to discuss their subjects. The chairman and secretary should be appointed from the committee members. Meetings should be held according to the set schedule throughout the year. The secretary should be assigned the responsibility of collecting samples and prices of material dealing with particular procedure or equipment.

The chairman then assigns the responsibility for investigation and development of problem under discussion, to a sub-group of master committee. Once this small group has reached the decision regarding the problem, the secretary writes up the material in accordance with predetermined format and submits it for the approval by master committee. After approval, the report should be distributed to the staff and pavilions.

QUESTIONS

1. What do you mean by O.P.D. ? What is its importance ?
2. Describe the location and lay out of O.P.D.
3. Write in short about "Out patient dispensing."
4. What are the various drug distribution systems for in-patients?
5. Write notes on the following:
   (i) Complete floor-stock system.
   (ii) Mobile dispensing unit.
   (iii) Labelling and inspection of floor stock drugs.
   (iv) Unit-dose dispensing system.
6. What are the advantages of satellite pharmacy services ?
7. Define central sterile supply services. Give a typical plan of central supply for medium sized hospital.
8. What are the duties of hospital pharmacist managing central sterile supply ?
9. Write a note on "Standardization Committee."

***

4

HOSPITAL MANUFACTURING

Hospitals are slowly moving to manufacture their medicinal requirement in the own premises. Hathi Committee has recommended the setting up of manufacturing units for I.V. fluids. Apart from sterile manufacture of large volume fluids and other parenterals, hospitals can manufacture non-sterile liquid oral preparations, externals and bulk preparations.

Factors affecting Economy of a Hospital: A hospital pharmacist should consider the following factors while keeping an adequate control over the manufacturing budget.

- **Manufacturing requirement:** The consumption rate for each item is calculated by reviewing the previous records and compared with present requirement.
- **Material requirement:** The raw material, packaging material and other materials required for manufacturing can be determined by various formulae.
- **Manufacturing staff:** Adequate number of technically competent and legally qualified pharmacists must be available in the manufacturing section.
- **Manufacturing capacity:** It depends on the availability of equipment and economy of a hospital to fulfill the requirement.
- **Manufacturing equipments:** The type and size of manufacturing equipment required in a hospital depends upon the manufacturing programme like the quantities to be produced, duration of production time, availability of personnel and availability of physical facilities.
- **Operating cost:** It includes both direct cost i.e. labour, cost of material etc. and indirect cost like maintenance of building, insurance policies etc.

Economic Considerations

Understanding the marketing environment of an industry or business or manufacturer is essential to size up the business. Various factors (social, ecological, legal, competitive) affect the marketing environment. One of the most important factors is the economic factor or environment of the business. Therefore, maximum economic considerations are required during the manufacture of a drug so as to give best quality with minimum cost.

The two principal ways in which the economic environment affects the business (manufacturing) are:

(i) Overall economic condition which affects the growth of the market and

(ii) Ability to raise finances to furnish the projects and growth plans.

It is true that we cannot alter the economic environment but we can certainly make reasonable judgements about its most likely future direction and make decisions that are consistent with those assumptions.

The following factors govern the economic consideration during the manufacture of a drug which affect decision to make or buy drug.

(i) Quality, (ii) Quantity, (iii) Cost and service.

(i) Quality: By comparing the quality of a drug produced in the hospital manufacturing unit and drug purchased from outside, one can decide whether to manufacture a drug or to buy it. If quality of purchased drug is better than manufactured one, then steps should be liken to improve the quality without increasing the manufacturing cost.

(ii) Quantity: Once the demand for a specific item is known, one can calculate the appropriate order quantities that will minimise overall purchasing costs. This is called as 'Economic Order Quantity'. Drugs which have relatively less demand or utilisation in a hospital are generally manufactured. Similarly those drugs required daily (of which the daily requirement is known) are also manufactured in the hospital. The break-even point analysis gives the quantity of drugs to be manufactured in the hospital on no profit or no loss basis.

(iii) Cost: By comparing of the cost of drugs bought from outside with those manufactured in the hospital, one can decide whether to make them in the hospital or buy them from outside. The determination of the cost of drug produced in the hospital should take into consideration the followings:

1. Cost of raw materials.
2. Processing cost
   - Building
   - Machine and furniture
   - Labour charges. etc.
3. Quality control charges.
4. Packaging cost.
5. Office cost: Printing, stationary, postage etc.

Service: Service provided by the supplier greatly influences 'to make or buy' decision. If the source of supply of raw material is assured, it results in efficient manufacturing of drugs in the hospital but if the supply is not assured, it affects or interrupts the clinical services of the hospital.

Controlling the Operating Process

Controlling the operation process is the success of any business. When operations go out of control, costs become excessive and delays occurs in patient (customer) service. The overall quality of care tends to suffer.

Product Control: There should be a strict control on the following:

1. Purchase of raw materials
   - (a) Purchase quantity decision
   - (b) Source of supply decision
   - (c) Purchase timing decision
   - (d) Purchase terms decision.
2. Manufacturing process control
   - (a) Selection of equipment
   - (b) Processing time
   - (c) Personnel requirements.
3. Control on quality of product.
4. Packaging control.

Estimation of Demand

There are three methods for estimation of demand for the drugs in hospital.

1. **Past Experience:** The experience and reviewing records of consumption of drugs in the past helps in deciding the requirement of drugs in future.
2. **Judgemental:** The clinical and pharmacy staff of the hospital gives an opinion about requirement of drugs (specific in the hospital for specific period) based on their experience.
3. **Casual Method:** By assessing the medical records of the hospital one can estimate the demand for a specific drug based on specific criterion. For example:

Demand of Drug	Criterion
1. Antibiotic drug	Number of patients admitted every month, for whom that specific drug was used.
2. Insulin	Number of patients with diabetes admitted every month.
3. Whole blood	Number of patients admitted in emergency wards.

QUESTIONS

1. Discuss the factors affecting economy of a hospital.
2. Discuss the factors affecting "make or buy decision".
3. Describe methods for estimation of demand of a drug in hospital.

***

5

STERILE MANUFACTURE

The sterile products are those dosage forms which are free from micro-organisms. These include parenteral preparations, ophthalmic preparations and irrigating fluids. The parenteral products are directly injected in the body.

Formulation

1. Vehicle: The most useful and commonly used vehicle for parenterals is water for injection (WFI). It should be free from ions and pyrogens. The water for injection must be prepared by distillation or reverse osmosis process and rendered free from ions by passing through an ion-exchange resin.

Sterile Water for Injection (SWFI): It is the water for injection sterilised and suitably packed. It contains no antimicrobial agent or other added substance.

The other non-aqueous vehicles which are used only for intramuscular injection are vegetable oils such as cotton seed oil, peanut oil, olive oil, glycerin, ethyl alcohol, propylene glycol etc.

2. Additives in parenterals: To maintain the quality of the injection until its time of administration, the additives used in parenterals should be of highest purity. The following additives are used in thc parenterals.

(a) To adjust the tonicity: Some injections need to be isotonic with blood or other body fluids. The tonicity of the solution is adjusted by using the substances like sodium chloride or borax or other substances which are compatible with other ingredients of the preparation. Various methods are used to estimate the amount of adjusting substances required to render a particular solution isotonic with plasma. e.g. Freezing point depression or sodium chloride equivalents.

(b) Antioxidants: To prevent the oxidative degradation of the parenteral products, antioxidants are added. The following substances are used as antioxidants for aqueous injections.

Sodium bisulphite

Sodium formaldehyde sulfoxylate

Thiourea, Acetone, Sodium metabisulphite

Sodium thiosulphate, ascorbic acid.

For oily injections: α-tocopherol, BHA, BHT and propyl gallate.

(c) Antimicrobials: Antimicrobials are used in the parenteral products to prevent the microbial growth especially in multidose container as during the withdrawal of the dose, the product may get contaminated. Hence to maintain the sterility of the product; the following antimicrobial agents are added in the adequate proportion. The antimicrobial agent should not be toxic and must be compatible with medicament.

Cresol	–	0.5%
Chlorocresol	–	0.2%
Benzalkonium chloride	–	0.001%
Chlorobutanol	–	0.5%
Phenylmercuric nitrate	–	0.002
Benzyl alcohol	–	1%

(d) Stabilizers: The stability of the preparation is most important factor in determining the quality of product. The parenterals, are more liable to decomposition through oxidation and hydrolysis. This can be prevented by adding antioxidants in the formulation or packing the product in an inert atmosphere of nitrogen or carbon dioxide.

The pH of the preparation is adjusted such that the decomposition by hydrolysis does not occur. The hydrolysis of the preparation can be avoided by replacing the water with other non-aqueous solvents. The use of EDTA in the preparation, complexes the metal ions and thus reduces the risk of degradation.

(e) Buffers: The use of buffering agents to maintain the pH of the parenteral product during its storage is important for preventing the degradation, by ionisation or by interaction of product with the material of the container. The generally used buffering systems are the citrates, phosphates, acetates of sodium, potassium, calcium and magnesium etc.

(f) Suspending, Emulsifying and Wetting Agents: To maintain the particle size of suspension and prevent flocculation and caking, the wetting agents used are Tween 80, Sorbiton trioleate. The suspending agents used are sodium CMC, Methyl Cellulose, Acacia, Gelatin, Polyvinyl Pyrrolidone (PVP) etc.

The most commonly used emulsifying agent for parenterals is lecithin.

Production Facilities

It is not only the quality of raw materials that gives best quality product but also the environment in which the product is manufactured and the manner of manufacturing process plays an important role in delivering the parenteral product.

Layout of Sterile Product Area

The entire area is divided into five different areas such as: clean up area, preparation area, aseptic area, quarantine area and packaging area.

1. Clean-up area: This area should withstand the effects of moisture, steam and detergents. The ceiling, floor and walls of this area should be constructed such that moisture will run off. For this purpose use of vinyl or epoxy sealing coat for finishing eliminates the holes in these surfaces. The area should be washed at regular intervals and properly exhausted. This area must be cleanable and precautions must be taken to prevent the growth of micro-organisms and collection of dust.

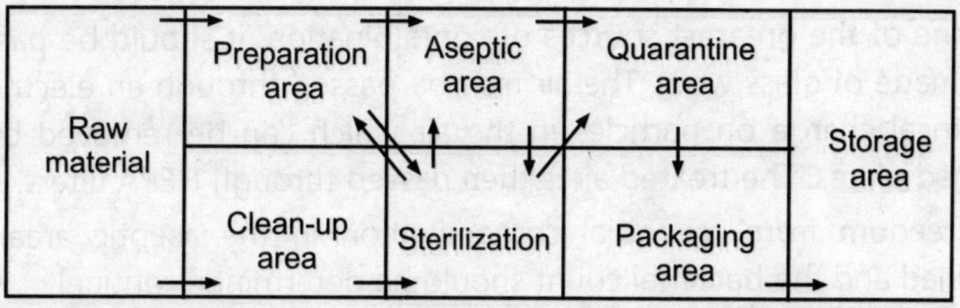

Fig. 5.1: Flow Diagram Showing Arrangement of Different Areas

2. Preparation area: It is also called as compounding area since the formula is compounded here. Although this area is not necessarily aseptic, a strict control over it than clean-up area is required. The means should be provided to control dust. The ceilings, walls and floor should be constructed similar to clean-up area. The cabinets and counters should be of stainless steel and these should be fitted in such a way that they should not catch dust.

3. Aseptic area: This area must be sealed so that it can be washed and sanitized with a disinfectant. All electricity, ventilation and utility service fittings should be in the walls or ceiling to eliminate joints where dust and dirt could accumulate. The mechanical equipment to be placed in this area should be kept within stainless steel cabinet.

Personnel should enter this area only through an airlock. The personnel must use sterile dresses, masks, caps and foot covers. There should be minimum movement in this area and the movement should be restricted during the filling hours. The air in the aseptic area should be free from fibres, dust and microbes. This can be achieved by use of High Efficiency Particulate Air (HEPA) filters. The HEPA filters are used in "laminar air flow" in which the air flows either horizontally or vertically along parallel lines. The velocity of 100 ft/min is the minimum effective air velocity.

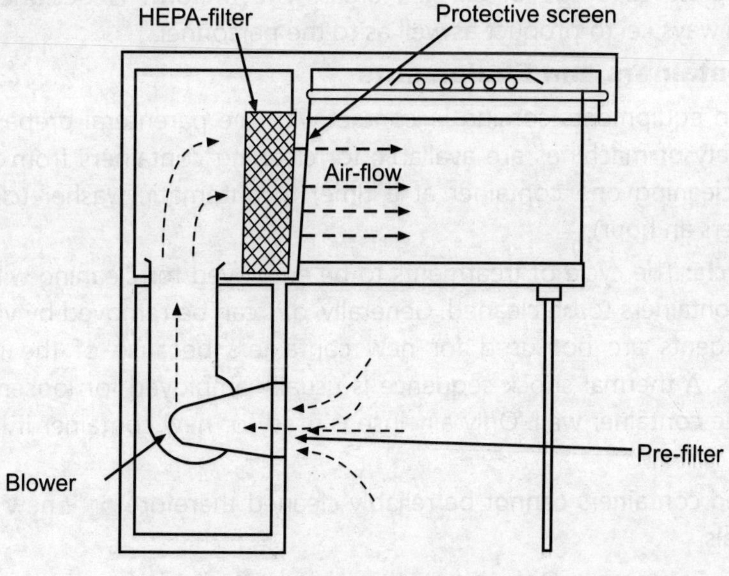

Fig. 5.2: Horizontal Laminar-flow

Since air is one of the greatest sources of contamination, it should be passed through a prefilter usually made of glass wool. The air may be passed through an electric device which induces an electrical charge on particles in the air which can be removed by attraction to oppositely charged plates. The treated air is then passed through HEPA filters.

To ensure freedom from microbial contamination in the aseptic area, it should be carefully maintained and the bacterial count should be determined routinely.

Personnel working in the aseptic area may contaminate the product under process. Hence personnel must wear sterile clothings, hoods, gloves and foot covers. The appropriate environmental control tests should also be performed to check the microbial contamination. The tests are based on the exposure of nutrient media plates to the environment and then incubating the plates for detecting the presence of microbes. Alternatively the sample of air can be taken through filters and placed on culture media and incubated for detection of microbes. All these are the different ways to reduce the particulate contamination and keep the environment of aseptic clean and room sterile for bulk manufacture and filling of intravenous products.

Personnel

The personnel selected for work in the preparation of parenteral product must be neat, orderly and reliable. They should be in good health and free from dermatological conditions. They must understand the unique requirements of aseptic procedures. They must receive instructions in the principles of aseptic processes.

Their uniform should be freshly laundered each day and sterile. The uniform consists of coveralls for both men and women, hoods for completely covering the hair, face masks and plastic boots. Sterile rubber gloves are required for most aseptic operations. Goggles may be required for complete coverage of all skin areas. The uniform is designed to give the protection in both ways i.e. to product as well as to the personnel.

Cleaning of Containers and Equipments

Containers and equipments coming in contact with the parenteral preparation must be cleaned well. Variety of machines are available for cleaning containers from single-jet tube (hand operated, cleaning one container at a time) to automatic washer (cleaning several thousand containers an hour).

Treatment cycle: The cycle of treatments to be employed for cleaning will vary with the condition of the containers to be cleaned. Generally, dirt can be removed by vigorous rinsing with water. Detergents are not used for new containers because of the risk of leaving detergent residues. A thermal shock sequence is usually employed for loosening the debris that adheres to the container wall. Only air rinse is used for new container if it is to be used for dry powder.

Previously used containers cannot be reliably cleaned therefore only new containers are used for parenterals.

Machinery for Containers: Different machineries are available for cleaning large number of containers. In one type, the jet tubes are arranged on arms like the spokes of a wheel, which rotate around a center post through which the treatments are introduced. An operator places the unclean containers on the jet tubes as they pass the loading point and removes the clean containers as they complete one rotation. The disadvantage of this machine is that it requires the individual handling of each container for loading and unloading. A type which overcomes this disadvantage is the rack-loading washer.

Rack-loading Washer: Racks are prepared to fit over the open ends of ampules or vials as they are found in shipping cartons. Carton is inverted to transfer the containers to washer without handling them individually. A battery of jet tubes is arranged to enter each container positioned in the rack. The clean containers may be removed in the rack and transferred to a box for dry heat sterilization and storage.

Handling of Containers: After cleaning, the wet containers are more liable to contaminate than dry ones. Hence these wet, rinsed containers should be protected by laminar air flow of clean air or covered within a stainless steel box and dry-heat sterilised.

Cleaning of Closures: The rubber closures are gently agitated in hot solution of 0.5% sodium pyrophosphate. The closures are then removed from solution and rinsed several times or continuously for prolonged time with water and finally with filtered WFI. The wet closures are then sterilized by autoclaving and stored in closed container until ready for use. If closures are required dry for use, then they are vacuum dried at temperature of 100°C. The equipment used for washing closures is usually an agitator or horizontal basket type automatic washing machine.

Equipment: Before cleaning, all equipment should be disassembled as much as possible to provide access to internal structures. The surfaces should be scrubbed thoroughly with a stiff brush using a detergent. Particularly the joints, crevices, screw threads and other structures where debris is apt to collect should be cleaned thoroughly. The surface of walls of stationary tanks and pipes should be exposed to a stream of clean steam to remove the residues. Large tanks should be protected from contamination after cleaning and should be rinsed thoroughly again with distilled water prior to use.

The cleaning is accomplished with scrubbing action of high pressure spray delivering hot detergent solution from tanks. Rubber tubing and rubber parts must be washed in the same way as rubber closures.

Requirements for the Manufacture of Parenteral Preparation

The following basic requirements are necessary for manufacturing parenteral preparation:

1. Strict sanitation is necessary throughout tile entire plant in order to prevent contamination. Masks and overheads should be used wherever necessary.
2. The preparation room should be air conditioned and tiled to keep it clean.
3. The filling and sealing rooms should be air conditioned under positive pressure with the provision of air locks.
4. The walls and floors should be tiled in such a way that permits easy spraying and washing with antiseptic solution. The tops of the benches should be of stainless steel or laminated plastic for easy washing.

5. There should be a provision of a separate room for sterilization, testing and drying.
6. The sufficient number of sterilizing lamps should be provided in the aseptic filling and sealing room to prevent contamination.
7. There should be provision for a separate room where labeling and packaging of product can be carried out.
8. The finished products should be stored in a separate clean and dry area.

Equipments

1. Storage equipment for ampoules and vials.
2. Ampoule washing and drying equipment.
3. Dust proof storage cabinets.
4. Water still and mixing tanks.

The material of the tanks or containers should not react with their contents.

5. Filtering equipments e.g. filter press.
6. Hot air sterilizer.
7. Benches for filling and sealing.
8. Filling and sealing unit.
9. Bacteriological filters e.g. Seitz filter, sintered glass filter, filter candles.
10. Inspection table.
11. Equipment for leak testing.
12. Benches for labelling and packing.
13. Storage equipments including refrigerators.

An area of 60 square meters is recommended for basic installations.

Preparation of the Bulk Solution

Usually facilities are provided for preparation of one batch at a time but whenever more than one batches are undergoing preparation at any one time, then precaution should be taken to ensure that cross contamination not occur. This does involves the appearance of physical barriers between various products. The effects of these physical barriers on air circulation must be taken into consideration. There should be easy access of injectable water. The chemicals to be used in the preparation of bulk solution should be delivered in proper containers. If injectable water is collected daily, then only one tank should be used for collection and it should not be allowed to stand for more than 4-6 hours. Sufficient space should be provided for inspection of tanks. The stirrers and heaters and scoops should be designed for easy cleaning and inspection. The problem of leakage of oil from bearings or gear box of stirrer usually occurs. The heating mechanism should be designed well to avoid local over heating. The metal surfaces coming in contact with the pharmaceutical product should be chosen with great care, especially the quality of welds and polish given to metals.

Filling of the Bulk Solution

During the filling of container with product, the precaution must be taken to prevent contamination since the product gets exposed to the environment, equipment and the operator until it is sealed in the dose container. Hence, this operation should be carried out in the aseptic filling area where maximum protection is provided by HEPA - filtered laminar flow air.

The liquid products are more readily subdivided uniformly and introduced into a container having a narrow mouth than the solid products. A means is provided for repetitively forcing a measured volume of the liquid through the orifice of a delivery tube which is introduced into the container.

During the filling the liquid product comes in intimate contact with the parts of machine, hence these must be constructed of non-reactive metal such as borosilicate glass or stainless steel. These parts should easily removable for cleaning and sterilization.

For filling of a small number of containers, hypodermic syringe and needle is used. Mechanically, operated instruments use a motor so that much faster filling rate can be achieved. By careful engineering the stroke of the syringe can be repeated and the setting of the machine is calibrated for the delivery.

For large volume solutions, the high speed fillers use bottle as the measuring device, transferring the bulk solution to the individual container.

Sealing: Sealing of the filled container should be done immediately to prevent the product contamination. The ampoules are sealed by melting a portion of glass neck with a fine jet of flame. Alternatively the fast sealing can be done by using oxygen flame. Sealing can be done by two methods:

(i) Tip seal (Bead seal) and

(ii) Pull seal

Tip Sealing	Pull Sealing
1. Tip of ampoule neck is heated to form a bead which closes the opening.	1. Little below the tip, the ampoule neck is heated. The tip is grasped firmly and pulled quickly with continuous rotation of ampoule neck over flame. The capillary tube thus formed twisted closed.
2. It is fast but not sure. Excessive heating may cause bubble on the tip.	2. It is slower but more sure.

Sometimes the air present, in the space above the product needs to be replaced by an inert gas, to avoid the decomposition. This is done by introducing a stream of inert gas (nitrogen, carbon dioxide) during or after the filling of product. Immediately sealing is done.

The vials and bottles are sealed by rubber closure (stopper). This must be done immediately after filling and with proper precautions to avoid contamination. Closures may be inserted aseptically with sterile forceps or directly by hands using sterile, rubber gloves. The rubber closures are held in place by means of aluminium caps. The caps cover the closure and are crimped under the tip of vial or bottle to hold them in place. Thus intact aluminium cap indicates that closure has not been removed at all and helps in protecting the contents.

These aluminium caps are available in three designs viz. single layered, double layered and tripple layered aluminium caps.

Sterilization

The parenteral product should be sterilized immediately after its sealing in final container (terminal sterilization). The sterilization is the process of making the product (object) free from microbes. Many products get adversely affected by temperature used for sterilization. Hence such products must be sterilized by non-thermal method such as filtration.

Sterilizing Method	Products
1. Dry heat (Hot air oven).	1. Dry solids that are not affected by high temperature and requiring longer heating period. Effective for glasswares and metalwares.
2. Moist heat under pressure (Autoclave).	2. Aqueous solutions or substances that can be penetrated by steam.
3. Ionizing radiation.	3. Dry solids such as streptomycin, polyvitamins, penicillin, catgut sutures.
4. Gaseous sterilization (Ethylene oxide).	4. Syringes, disposable needles, administration sets, plastic and stainless steel equipment.
5. Bacteria proof filtration.	5. Thermolabile products.
6. Lyophilisation.	6. Preservation of human tissue.

The effectiveness of any sterilization method should be checked from time to time. For this purpose biological indicators are useful for ascertaining the effectiveness of the method.

Evaluation of Parenterals

The following tests are used for the evaluation of parenteral products.

1. Sterility Test: The sterility test does not signify that product is sterile but indicates a probable sterility of batch of products. The I.P. describes this test. The product to be tested is transferred aseptically in sterile nutrient media and incubated for specific period of time at an optimum temperature. If living microbes are present, the growth takes place on the media and if absent then no growth is observed on the media. The test should be carried out under aseptic conditions. Product containing bacteriostatic agent may give a false negative test. Hence such product is diluted to make bacteriostatic agent ineffective and then the test is carried out. Products containing antimicrobial drugs e.g. Penicillin, sulfa drugs have to be tested in presence of antagonistic materials e.g. penicillin in presence of penicillinase and sulfa drugs with PABA.

The nutrient medium must be sterile and able to produce microbial growth. If test for sterility gives negative results (no microbial growth) then the product is considered sterile but the test is repeated again to make sure. If the test gives positive results (i.e. microbial growth), the product is non-sterile and test is repeated twice or thrice to check for accidental contamination. If again test fails then product is non-sterile.

2. Pyrogen Test: Pyrogens are metabolic products of living or dead micro-organisms which cause an increase in body temperature after injection. Chemically pyrogens are lipopolysaccharides soluble in water but insoluble in organic solvents. Since they are water soluble, they can not be removed by autoclaving or filtration.

The USP pyrogen test requires healthy mature rabbits as test animals to determine the absence or presence of pyrogens in the products. Three rabbits are used and receive 10 ml of the test solution per kg of body weight by injection into an ear vein, completing the injection within 10 min. The rectal temperature is recorded at 1, 2 and 3 hours after the injection. The sample passes the test if at no time during this three hours period after injection, the temperature of any rabbit rises by more than 0.6°C or the sum of the rise in temperature for three rabbits exceeds 1.4°C. If these limits are exceeded the test is expanded to include five additional rabbits after which the requirement for absence of pyrogen states that no more than three rabbits each exhibits a temperature rise of less than 0.6°C and the total temperature rise for all eight rabbits is 3.7°C or less.

LAL (Limulus Amebocyte Lysate) test is another method for detection of pyrogens. The sample solution to be tested is combined with lysate of blood cells (amebocytes) of horseshoe crab. If pyrogens or any endotoxin is present in the sample, it will get coagulated with proteins of the blood cells and result in the formation of gel.

3. Leaker Test: It is performed by producing a negative pressure within an incompletely sealed ampoule while the ampoule is entirely submerged in a deep coloured dye solution. A 1% methylene blue solution is usually employed. After releasing the vacuum, the coloured dye solution enters the incompletely sealed ampoules.

Another test frequently employed is to simply autoclave the ampoules in a dye bath. A modification of this test is to remove them from autoclave while hot and quickly dip in a cool bath of dye solution. After carefully rinsing the dye solution from outside, colour from the dye will be visible within a leaker i.e. a leaking ampoule is called as leaker and all the leakers have to be discarded.

4. Clarity Test: The presence of particles in solution particularly if injected intravenously is harmful since it can produce emboli in vital organs of the body. To prevent the distribution and use of such parenteral products, it is necessary to perform the clarity test. The basic mechanism of clarity testing consists of human visual inspection under good light against black and white background. This helps in visualisation of transparent particles against black background and coloured particles against white background. This visual inspection has its own limitations such as individual variation of visual acuity, emotional state, eye strain and fatigue. Visual inspection will not detect particles smaller than 50 μm.

USP has established microscopic test method for large volume parentarals. It consists of filtering a measured sample of solution through membrane filter under ultraclean conditions and then counting the particles on the surface of filter under a microscope.

Limits: Not more than 50 particles/ml of 10 μm and larger in size and not more than 5 particles/ml of 25 μm and larger in size.

Many electronic particle counters are available that use the light scattering principle to count particles in a liquid sample. Coulter counter is also useful in detecting the particulate matter. In addition to above tests, the National Institute of Health requires most biological products to undergo routine safety testing in animals.

QUESTIONS

1. Define sterile product.
2. What do you mean by WFI, SWFI and BWFI ?
3. Write a short note on "Additives in Parenterals."
4. Describe the layout of sterile product area.
5. Write in brief about the aseptic area for the manufacture of sterile products.
6. Give the different methods of sterilization for parenterals.
7. Describe the various production facilities required for manufacture of sterile product.
8. Write a note on "Filling and sealing of parenteral solution.
9. Describe the following tests for evaluation of parenteral solution.
   (a) Sterility test (c) Leaker test
   (b) Pyrogen test (d) Clarity test.
10. What do you know about "Personnel" in the manufacture of sterile products ?
11. Give the basic requirements for the manufacture of parenteral preparation.

***

6

NON-STERILE MANUFACTURE

Manufacture of Tablet

Tablets are not containing solely the drug but it also contains an added substance (additives) to make the powder more compressible and increase fluidity during manufacture.

The fluidity is required to enhance the flow of powder from hopper to 'die' cavity uniformly to get the tablets of uniform weight. Fluidity can be increased by incorporating a glidant (e.g. fumed silicon-dioxide in proportion of 0.01%).

Compressibility is the ability of powder to form a compact mass after applying pressure. The granulation of powder increases the compressibility

Methods of Granulation

The current methods of granulation are:

(i) Wet granulation,

(ii) Dry granulation, and

(iii) Direct compression.

(i) Wet granulation: It is widely used method for production of compressed tablets. The ingredients of the formulation are weighed accordingly and blended. Then a damp mass is prepared by adding a liquid binder (binding agent) e.g. starch, various gums and cellulose derivatives (methyl cellulose, carboxy methyl cellulose, microcrystalline cellulose), gelatine. The damp mass is then screened into pellets or granules. (number '6' or '8' mesh screen is used). The granules are spread on large pieces of paper in a shallow tray and dried. The granules are dried in thermostatically controlled drying cabinets. Fluid bed driers are used for this purpose. The dried granules are then passed through a screen of smaller mesh than that used for preparing original granulation. (It is called as dry screening) After dry screening, a lubricant in the dry form is added to the granules so that each granule is covered with lubricant. The quantity of lubricant depends on tableting operation and ranges from 0.1% of weight of granules to 5%. Various types of tablet presses or tablet machines are used to compress the tablet.

(ii) Dry granulation (Slugging): The granules are prepared by screening previously prepared large compact masses (slugs) of the mixture. It is applicable to substances which have cohesive properties and those which can't be granulated by above method.

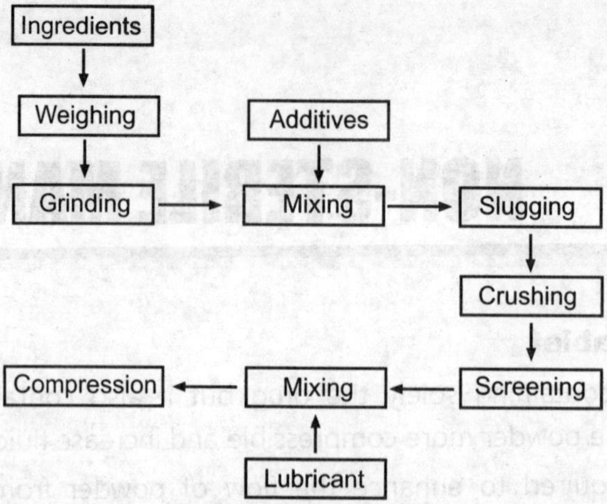

(iii) Direct compression: Some chemical substances like potassium chloride, potassium iodide, ammonium chloride possess free flowing as well as cohesive properties. Hence these can be compressed directly without granulation.

After compression of tablets, they are deducted to remove traces of powder adhering to tablets surface. The deducted tablets are then subjected to different types of coating.

Requirements of equipments for the manufacturing of pills and compressed tablets

(a) **Granulating section:** Disintegrator, powder mixer, mass mixer, granulator, thermostatically controlled ovens.

(b) **Tableting section:** Tablet machine (single punch or rotary), pill machine, punch and dies storages cabinet, tablet counter.

(c) **Coating section:** Jacketed kettle, steam, gas or electrically heated for preparing solution. Coating pan, polishing pan, heater and exhaust system.

The coating section should be made dust free and suitable exhaust should be provided to remove excess powder and the fumes resulting from solvent evaporation. An area of 30 square metres for each of the above three sections is recommended for basic installations.

Manufacture of Powders: Powder, as a pharmaceutical dosage form, is a mixture of finely divided drugs (obtained from vegetable origin) and/or chemicals in dry form.

Various types of mills and pulvarizers are used to reduce powder fineness.

Mixing of Powders: It is best to reduce the particle size of individual ingredients before weighing and blending. The powders are then mixed together by different methods such as as spatulation, trituration, shifting and mechanical mixers.

The following equipments are recommended for the manufacture of powders in Drugs and Cosmetics Rules, 1945.

1. Disintegrator,
2. Mixer,
3. Sifter,
4. Stainless steel vessels and scoops,
5. Filling equipment.

A suitable exhaust system should be provided. Workers should be provided with suitable masks during operation. An area of 30 square metres is required.

The mixing by spatulation and trituration is for making powders on a small scale basis, whereas sifters and mixers are used for large scale manufacturing.

These mixed powders are then packed according to the need, in bulk form or in divided form. The bulk powders are usually antacid powders, dental cleansing powders, medicated powder, powders for vaginal use (douche powders).

In case of divided powder, the powder is divided into individual units depending on dose or amount to be used at single time.

The powder papers used for wrapping individually divided powder are of different types:

1. Simple bond paper, white or coloured,
2. Parchment paper,
3. Waxed paper, transparent, waterproof paper,
4. Glazed transparent paper.

Capsules: These are dosage forms in which the medicament is enclosed within a hard or soft gelatine shell.

Soft gelatin capsules are formed, filled and sealed in one manufacturing operation and may contain solid powder or oily liquids, solutions, emulsions and pastes.

The hard gelatine capsule shells are manufactured from a mixture of gelatine, sugar and water and are clear, colourless and essentially tasteless. These are manufactured in two parts viz. capsule body and cap. The shells are produced by mechanically dipping the pegs of desired shape into melted gelatine mixture maintained at a constant temperature. The pegs affixed to plates are submerged in melted gelatine mixture to a desired depth and time. The plate with pegs are then slowly lifted up and dried by a flow of temperature and humidity controlled air. Different varieties of capsules can be prepared. e.g. coloured opaque capsules may be produced by adding colorant and opacity producing substance such as titanium dioxide to a gelatine mixture.

Planning: The amount of formula (quantities of drug and diluent) to be prepared depends on the number of capsules.

The selection of capsule size is best done during the formulation, since the amount of materials required depends on the size of capsule. If formulation does not require diluent for adjusting the bulk, then size of capsule can be selected after developing and preparing the formulation.

Filling of Capsules

The pharmacist that regularly prepares capsules in the hospital uses hand operated capsule filling machine.

The following equipments are recommended in Drugs and Cosmetics Rules 1945 for manufacture of capsules.

1. Mixing and blending equipment,
2. Capsule filling units,
3. Capsule counters.

An area of 25 square metres is recommended for capsule filling. The room should be air conditioned and dehumidified whenever necessary and suitable exhaust system should also be provided.

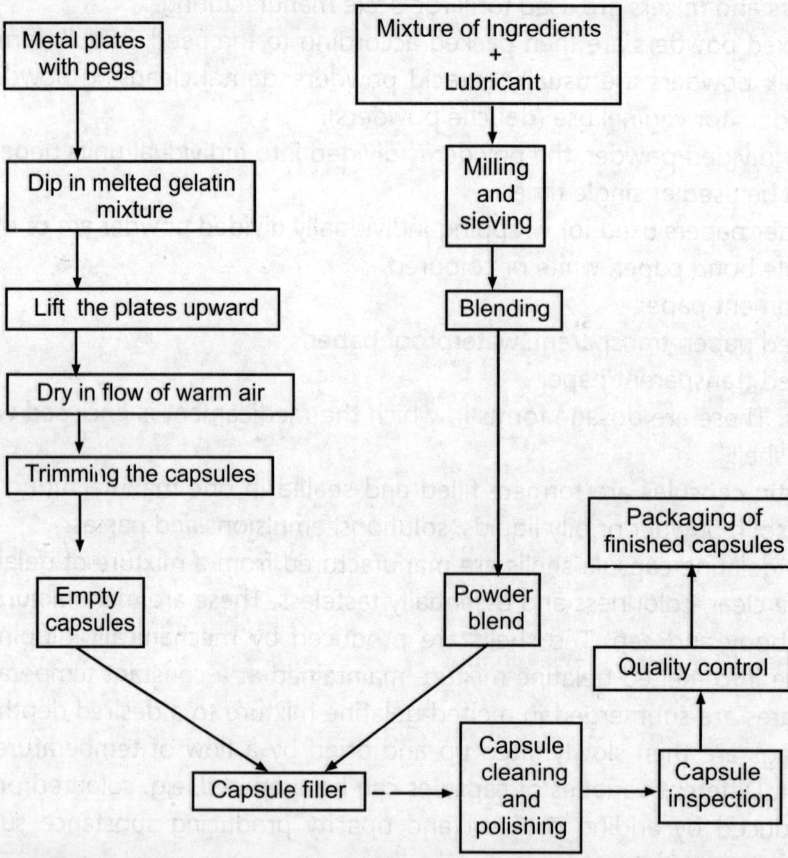

The manufacturing capacity of the capsule filling machine varies and depends on its type, whether manual, semi-automatic or automatic.

The U.S.P. prescribes the following standards for the capsules:

(i) Content uniformity.

(ii) Weight variation.

Soft Gelatin Capsules

Preparation: These are prepared from gelatin to which glycerin or sorbitol is added to render it elastic. The capsules are prepared either by plate method or by rotory die process machine.

Plate Method: On bottom plate of mold a warm sheet of gelatin is placed and the liquid medicament is evenly poured. Another sheet of prepared gelatine then placed on top and kept in position. The mold is then pressed to form capsules. The capsules are removed and then washed with solvent.

Rotary Die Method: In this method, two distinct ribbons are formed by the machine from liquid gelatine. These two ribbons are brought together between two rotating dies. Simultaneously when two ribbons form a pocket (due to die cavities) a filler material of specified quantity is injected in the pocket and it is sealed by application of pressure and heat in the machine. According to the design of die cavity, the soft gelatine capsules may be prepared in different shapes.

Facilities Required for Manufacture of Tablets, Powders and Capsules

Tablets, powders and capsules need to be manufactured in a controlled environment. This space should provide areas of access through which materials and equipment can enter or leave through one side and personnel through the other. There should be areas where personnel can change into working cloths and for cleaning the equipment prior to it entrance into the working area. Each access zone or area should be equipped with self closing doors. The working area should be ventilated in such a way that air entering it is passes through a purification system. Routine environmental inspection should be undertaken to confirm that conditions as per the required standards.

A locked cupboard should be provided for the storage of dry products. The dust extraction point should be provided at each weighing station.

Granulation: If materials are to be mixed by hands, then mixing tray should have extended sides and stainless steel scoops should be provided for removal of material without significant loss. In case of machines, the equipment should be easily cleaned between the batches. Equipment should not allow lubricating oils to gain contact with the product. The machine should be employed with safety requirements.

Vacuum cleaners and dedusting unit should be provided for the dust extraction. Controls must be exercised to prevent contamination of water supply.

The sinks provided for washing should be sufficiently deep and with rounded corners.

A facility of weighing the product at various stages should be provided.

Dry Blending: Dust control and personnel protection by suitable clothing of operator is essential.

Compression: During this stage, facilities of measuring thickness, hardness and weight variation should be provided adjacent to the machine. Other tests of disintegration and friability are preformed in Q.C. laboratory. Before the start and at the final stage of compression, Q.C. staff must be informed for the approval of the batch.

Manufacture of Liquid Orals

The liquid formulations are meant for internal as well as external use:

(i) Internal use: Oral solutions elixirs, linctuses, syrups, mixtures, drops.

(ii) External use: Lotions, liniment, EENT preparations, enemas, douches, inhalation liquids.

Planning

Solutions: Simple solution are prepared by dissolving the solute in the solvent or solvent mixture. Colourants, flavourants, stabilizers and preservatives may be added to these solutions.

Syrups: These are concentrated aqueous preparations of sugar and medicinal substance with or without added flavouring agent.

Most syrups contain sugar (usually sucrose), preservative, colouring agent, flavouring agent and may be solubilizers and stabilizers.

Preparation of Syrup

These can be prepared by the following methods - Solution of the ingredients.

(i) With the aid of heat.

(ii) By agitation without use of heat.

(iii) By addition of sucrose to a prepared medicated liquid

(iv) By precolation of sucrose.

Preparation of Elixirs

These are prepared by simple method of solution by agitation and/or by the admixture of two or more liquid ingredients. The water soluble ingredients are dissolved in water and alcohol soluble ingredients are dissolved in alcohol and then the aqueous solution is added to alcoholic solution. After complete mixing of two solutions, volume of mixture is adjusted with specified solvent. If mixture becomes cloudy, allow it to stand for few hours and filter it. The glycerin, syrup, sorbitol in the elixir enhances its stability.

Requirements

The following equipments are recommended in the Drugs and Cosmetics Rules, 1945 for the manufacture of Syrups, Elixirs and Solutions.

1. Mixing and Storage tanks.
2. Portable mixer.
3. Filter press or metafilter or sparklet filter.
4. Vacuum or gravity filter.
5. Water still or Deioniser.

The area required for the manufacture of these is 30 square metres.

"Manufacture of Externals"

Preparation of Ointment: The ointment may either be medicated or non-medicated. The non-medicated ointments are the ointment bases and are used as emmolient or lubricants or as vehicle in preparation of medicated ointments.

Ointment bases: These are of four types:

(a) Absorption bases, (b) Water soluble bases,

(c) Hydrocarbon bases, (d) Water miscible bases.

Absorption bases: These are of two types:

(i) Non-emulsified: These bases absorb water to produce water in oil (w/o) emulsion. These consists of mixture of an emulsifying agent with one or more paraffins.

E.g.: Wool fat, Wool alcohol, Bees wax and Cholesterol.

Bees wax and cholesterol are included in some ointment bases to increase its water absorbing power.

(ii) Emulsion bases (w/o emulsions): These are already w/o emulsions, which permit incorporation of small quantities of water or aqueous solution.

E.g. Hydrous wool fat (lanolin), Cold cream.

Water soluble bases: These are developed from polyethylene glycols. These bases have the advantage of being non-occlusive, miscible with exudates, non-staining and easily removable by washing. These are non-toxic and non-irritant to skin.

Disadvantage of these bases in that they reduce the activity of antimicrobial substances like phenols, quaternary ammonium compounds and hydroxybenzoates.

E.g.

1. Bentonite - 10	II. Gelatin - 15
Glycerin - 10	Glycerin - 35
Water - 70	Water - 35

Hydrocarbon - Bases: (Water Insoluble bases)

These bases absorb very little water from skin exudates or formulations and do not get absorbed by skin. These form water proof film and thus avoid water loss. By improving the hydration of skin, enhances the absorption of medicament.

E.g. Soft paraffin, Hard paraffin and Liquid paraffin, Paraffin ointment B.P. and Petrolatum (White and yellow).

These are used mainly for their emmolient effect and are difficult to wash off.

Water miscible bases: Though these can emulsify large quantities of water they are immiscible with an excess of water. These can be easily removed after use. These consists of paraffins and o/w emulsifying agents.

E.g. Emulsifying wax	-	30%
Liquid paraffin	-	20%
White soft paraffin	-	50%

Advantages of these bases are easy removal from skin, miscibility with exudates of skin, good contact with skin.

The ointments are prepared by two methods viz. fusion method and incorporation method.

(a) Fusion Method

The ingredients are melted together and cooled with constant stirring. Heat labile and volatile ingredients are added at the end. On large scale the process is carried out in large steam-jacketed kettles. Medicated ointments and ointments containing bees wax, stearyl alcohol and paraffins are manufactured by this method.

(b) Incorporation Method

The ingredients of ointment are mixed together by mortar and pestle or by ointment slab and spatula.

Solid: When small amount of powder is to be added, it is levigated by mixing with insoluble solvent to form a fine dispersion. After levigation it is incorporated in small amount of ointment bases and the process is repeated until whole of ointment base is incorporated.

Liquids: Hydrophilic or water absorbable base is suitable for absorption and incorporation of aqueous solutions. If an aqueous preparation is to be added in the hydrophobic base, then a portion of base is replaced by hydrophilic base in which the aqueous preparation is added and then diluted with original base. Small volumes of alcoholic solutions can be added well to emulsion bases.

For large scale manufacturing, roller type ointment mills are convenient. Hobart type mixers are useful for cream type of bases. The triple roller mill is preferable due to its greater output

The cross section of the triple roller mill is shown in Fig. 6.1. The three rollers arranged in contact with each other rotate at different speeds, increasing from left to right. The right sided roller takes the ointment from left side and finally the scraper collects the ointment. Due to friction, the temperature of rollers increases which is prevented by water-jacketing the rollers. The triple roller mill can be sterilised by 5% aqueous phenol solution or ultraviolet light.

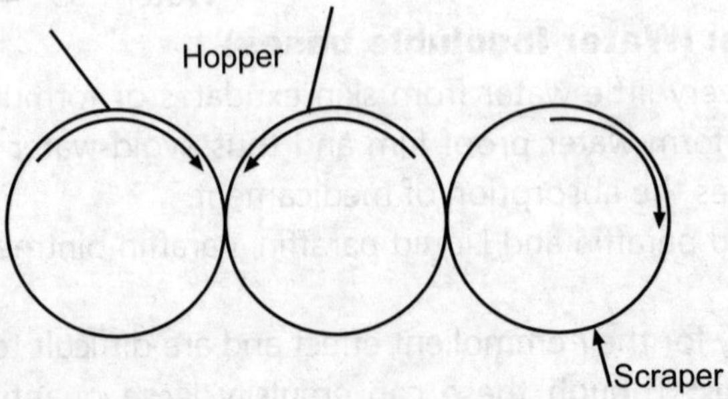

Fig. 6.1

Other Additives in Ointment

(i) Preservatives: These are not required in anhydrous ointments but essential for ointments with aqueous components. Organic mercurials, quaternary ammonium compounds, benzalkonium chloride, benzoic acid are generally used.

(ii) Antioxidants: e.g. Butylated Hvdroxy Anisole (BHA), Butylated Hydroxy Toluene (BHT) and Ethyl or propyl Gallates.

EMULSIONS

While developing the formulation of an emulsion the choice of aqueous phase, oil phase and emulsifying agent in their correct proportion is important

The relative proportions of oil and water phase depends on the dosage requirement or the consistency and stability of the emulsion. The oil phase is selected on the basis of compatibility, stability, toxicity and desired consistency. Generally, edible oils are used.

Type of Emulgent:

Emulgents are of three types:

1. Synthetic emulgents:

Anionic surfactants - e.g. sodium, potassium or ammonium salts of oleic and stearic acid. They produce o/w emulsion. Calcium salts of fatty acids, triethanolamine soap, sodium lauryl sulphate.

Cationic surfactants - Cetrimide.

Non-ionic surfactants - e.g Glycol and Glycerol esters, Sorbitan ester and polysorbates.

2. Natural products:

e.g. Acacia, tragacanth, wool fat, bees wax.

3. **Finely divided Solids:** e.g. Clays, Bentonite, Aluminium magnesium silicate, Silica gel.

The 'hydrophile-lipophile balance' (HLB) can be used to select appropriate emulsifying agent for a particular system. Other additives in emulsion are antimicrobial agents, antioxidants and viscosifying agents. Following machines are used for manufacture of emulsion.

1. Mixers,
2. Homogenisers,
3. Colloid mills, and
4. Ultrasonic emulsifiers.

Mixer and homogenisers are especially used for suspensions. Colloid mill is used for reducing the globule size. Preformed coarse emulsion is fed into the mill and the globule size is reduced by shearing action.

Requirements

The Drugs and Cosmetics Rules, 1945 recommended the following equipment for the manufacture of ointments and emulsions.

1. Mixing tanks
2. Kettle, steam, gas or electrically heated.
3. A suitable power-driven mixer.
4. Storage tanks or pots.
5. A colloid mill or a suitable emulsifier.
6. A triple roller mill or an ointment mill.
7. Liquid filling equipment.
8. Jar or tube filling equipment.

An area of 30 square metres is recommended for the basic installations.

Facilities

The risk of microbial growth is greater in aqueous system than other. The sources of contamination during manufacture and filling of these products are numerous such as:

1. Stortage of water in tanks which are not adequately cleaned.
2. Badly designed piping system for the supply of distilled water at the site of use.
3. The manufacturing equipments has cavities where the water gets trapped resulting in improper cleaning.
4. Insufficient space and facility for cleaning and storage of equipment.
5. Use of contaminated disinfectants.
6. Inadequate ventilation at the site of manufacture.
7. Overcrowding of product and personnel.
8. Improper hygienic procedures for manufacturing of the product.
9. Inadequate facilities for the control of manufacturing process.

All these risks should be avoided while providing the facilities for the manufacture.

The manufacturing should be carried out in a controlled environment provided with access zones.

Some products require bulk manufacturing in clean conditions followed by sterilization of the bulk product by membrane filtration.

The sterilised product is then filled aseptically into previously sterilised containers.

Sometimes the two parts of the product need to be sterilized separately and then blended or homogenized aseptically and then filled aseptically. The provision of continuous stirring and warming of the product is essential during the filling of the product.

The bulk manufacturing area should be separated from the filling area by a floor to ceiling physical barrier.

The environment may be kept pleasant by keeping the physical barrier half glassed which also helps in easier supervision.

A facility must be provided for the safe storage of bulk product awaiting for QC approval prior to its filling.

The filling area should be inspected by a responsible person who would be incharge of removing all items of previous batch and confirms by signature. The adequate facility for washing the bottles and closures should be provided. The rinsing and washing process should expose the bottles to powerful jets of hot aqueous detergent solution followed by cold water.

The containers and closures require the pre-treatment before filling. Hence the filling zone must be adjacent to the pre-treatment area.

After washing, the containers and closures should be dried in the drying oven.

Suppositories

The most important aspect in formulation of suppositories is the selection of proper base. There are two main types of suppository bases. (1) Fatty/oleaginous base (2) Water soluble/water miscible base.

1. **Fatty or Oleaginous Bases:** e.g. Theobroma oil (Cocoa butter).

Theobroma oil is a mixture of glyceryl esters of stearic palmitic and oleic acids.

Advantages

1. Non-irritating.
2. Melts at 30-36°C.
3. Miscible with many ingredients.

Disadvantages

1. On cooling it does not contract sufficiently and a problem of adherence to mould occurs.
2. Depending on the temperature of melting and speed of cooling, the oil solidifies in different crystalline forms called as polymorphism. Such crystals formed solidify at lower temperature than the oil and thus may be in liquid state at room temperature.

3. It may become rancid on storage.
4. The water absorbing ability of the oil is poor.
5. Melting point may be reduced by ingredients.
6. It is expensive.

These disadvantages of theobroma oil can be overcome by synthetic hard fat bases e.g. Hydrogenated Palm Kernel oil.

2. **Water Soluble Bases:** Two main types of bases are:
(i) Glycerogelatin base, and (ii) Polyethylent, glycols base.

(i) Glycerogelatin base:

It is used in the preparation of vaginal suppositories.

Disadvantages

1. Unpredictable solution time.
2. The hygroscopic nature of the base requires that it be protected from heat and moisture.
3. The dehydrating effect of the base causes irritation to the rectal or vaginal mucosa.
4. Lubrication of the mould is required for removal of suppository from mould.
5. Preservatives are required in the formulation to prevent microbial contamination which results in incompatability.
6. The suppositories have a laxative effect.

(ii) Polyethylene Glycol Base (PEG base)

These materials have a wide range of melting points and solubilities. Hence it is possible to prepare the suppositories of varying heat stability and dissolution rates.

These are chemically polymers of ethylene oxide and water prepared to various chain lengths and molecular weights. The number indicates the average molecular weight of that polymer.

E.g.

I.	PEG 1000 - 75%	II.	96%
	PEG 4000 - 25%		4%

Advantages

1. The base contracts slightly on cooling. Therefore does not require lubrication of mould.
2. No laxative effect.
3. The base gives suppositories a clean, smooth appearance.
4. These bases have good solvent properties.
5. The base dissolves in the body at higher temperature and thus gives slow release action of the medicament.

Disadvantages

1. Due to good solvent properties, the drug may get retained in the base resulting in poor bioavailability.
2. These bases are incompatible with plastics and this limits the choice of container.
3. The hygroscopic nature of the base may cause irritation to the mucosa.

Additives of Suppository

Antioxidants and preservatives which are required for the suppository and are chosen on the basis of their compatibility.

The emulgents such as wool fat, emulsifying wax, polysorbates are included in the formulation to facilitate incorporation of aqueous solutions.

Preparation of Suppositories

The suppositories are prepared by three methods:

I. Moulding II. Compression and III. Hand rolling.

I. Preparation of Suppositories by Moulding

This method is commonly used. The base material is melted and the required amount of medicament is dissolved or suspended in it. Then the melt is poured into the mould and allowed to cool to form the suppositories. Suppositories on setting are removed from mould.

Generally, molds are made up of stainless steel, aluminium, brass or plastic. In the machine moulding process, the operations of pouring, cooling and removal from moulds are carried out on an automated machine. The output of rotary machine is about 3000-6000 suppositories per hour.

Lubrication of Moulds: For easy removal of suppository from the mould, lubrication of the mould with mineral oil is essential.

Calibration of Moulds: Calibration of the mould with the base is necessary for all moulds to determine the exact capacity of particular mould. This figure is used for calculating the quantities.

Method for Determination of Displacement Value

The general mold of 1 g or 15 grain is used.

1. Prepare and weigh six suppositories of base only.
   Suppose its weight is 'A' g.
2. Prepare and weigh '6' suppositories of base containing 30% medicament.
   Suppose its weight is 'B' g.
3. Calculate the amount of base 'C' g and drug 'D' g in these six suppositories.
   C = 70% 'B'
   D = 30% 'B'
4. Therefore the amount of base displaced by drug

$$Dg = A - Cg$$

$$\text{Displacement value} = \frac{D}{A - C}$$

For Example

1. Weight of six suppositories of bane only = 8.0 g (A).
2. Weight of six suppositories containing 30% drug = 10 g (B)
3. Quantity of base = 70% of 10 = 7.0 g (C)

Quantity of drug = 30% of 10 = 3.0 g (D)

∴ Base displaced by 3.0 g of drug (D) 8.0 − 7.0 g = 1.0 g

∴ Displacement value of the drug = $\frac{3.0}{1.0}$ = 3

The list of displacement values with respect to bases of various 40 drugs are given in the literature.

II. Preparation of Suppositories by Compression

The suppository base and medicaments are mixed together and the mass is then forced by pressure into the moulds of the machine. On small scale, the mortar and pestle is used whereas on large scale it requires mixers and warmed vessels.

The method is suitable for thermolabile substances and for insoluble medicaments in the base. It is unsuitable for glycerogelatin base suppositories.

A special machine is required for preparation of suppositories, in which the mixed mass is forced on one side of machine through the cylinder and on other side, the moulds or die cavities are present. These die cavities get filled with this mass. A movable end plate supports the back of these die cavities so that when this plate is removed and additional force is applied on insertion side of machine, the formed suppositories from die cavities are ejected. The movable plate is returned to its position and the process is repeated to produce continuously the suppositories.

III. Preparation of Suppositories by Hand Rolling and Shaping

The pharmacist prefers this method in the hospital, when small number of units need to be prepared in cocoa butter base.

The medicament is mixed with cocoa-butter and triturated well to achieve uniform distribution and form a plastic mass. This plastic mass is then formed into ball with the hand. The ball is rolled into the cylinder of specific length with a steel spatula. The cylinder is divided into equal segments (about 1 inch) with sharp blade. With the help of fingers or spatula, one end of the segment is tapered to the desired shape.

Requirements

The Drugs and Cosmetics Rules 1945 recommend the following equipment for the manufacture of suppositories.

1. Mixing and pouring equipment.
2. Molding equipment.

An area of 20 square metres is recommended for the basic installations.

Bulk Concentrates: Usually the solutions and semisolids are compounded in bulk and as concentrates. The bulk compounded liquid orals include syrups, elixirs, suspensions and emulsions. The semisolids which are compounded in bulk include emulsions and ointments.

QUESTIONS

1. Describe the facilities required for the manufacture of compressed tablets.
2. Describe different methods of granulation for tablets.
3. Give the methods of manufacture of soft gelatine capsules.
4. Name the equipments required for the manufacture of
   (i) Tablet
   (ii) Liquid orals
   (iii) Ointment and emulsion.
5. Describe the facilities required for manufacture of ointment and emulsions.
6. Describe the production planning for ointments.
7. Write in short about:
   (i) Ointment bases
   (ii) Suppository bases.
8. Describe the preparation of suppositories by moulding.
9. Write in short about manufacture of powders.

***

7

STORES PURCHASES AND INVENTORY CONTROL

Purchase and inventory control of pharmaceuticals is of great importance in running the hospital pharmacy successfully. The word inventory is defined as – "an itemized list of goods with their estimated worth; specifically an annual account of stock taken in any business".

The pharmacist incharge is responsible for specifications both as to quality and source for purchase of all drugs, chemicals, antibiotics, biologicals and pharmaceutical preparations used in the treatment of patients.

Drug Storage and Inventory Control

Storage of drugs is an important aspect of the total drug control system. Proper environmental control must be maintained wherever drugs and supplies are stored. The storage area must be secure and the equipments used to store drugs should be constructed such that drugs are accessible only to designated personnel. Safety of storage of drugs is also important and poisons and in flammable compounds must be stored safely. Externals should be stored separately from internal medications.

Proper control is required such as expiry dates of drugs stored in all locations must be considered and accordingly the stock rotated as required. A method should be established to detect outdated; deteriorated, recalled drugs. It should include monthly audit of all medication storage areas.

Role of Pharmacist in Purchasing (procurement) of Drugs

The drugs for hospital use may be purchased as follows:

1. Directly from manufacturer.
2. Directly from wholesaler.
3. From either manufacturer or wholesaler by bid.
4. From local retail pharmacy (In emergency only).
5. By contract purchase arrangement with manufacturer.
6. By contract purchase through a hospital purchase bureau or corporation.

In case of bid purchasing, when bids from manufacturers are opened, the lowest bidder should receive the purchase order, however he should assure that the hospital gets the best quality of merchandise (item). On the other hand, if bidding is by vendors then the hospital or local laboratory must make arrangements for analytical and clinical testing of samples.

The hospital pharmacist should discuss with the purchasing agent (officer) and choose the method for purchasing the drugs. In addition he also performs the following duties:

1. Maintains a list of names, addresses and telephone numbers of drug manufacturers, wholesalers and their local agents.
2. Prepares "Request for purchase" forms.
3. Prepares detailed specifications required for drugs, chemicals and biologicals.
4. Prepares "Receiving memo" if drugs are received directly by the pharmacy.
5. Prepares "Return Goods Memo" whenever applicable.

Role of "Purchasing Officer" in purchasing of Drugs

Personnel

The role of a purchasing officer may vary from small hospital to large hospital. In small hospital, the function of purchasing may be handled by administrator or his assistant or store-keeper. Due to lack of time or pressure of other duties, an individual gives less importance to this function. Whereas in large hospitals, one or more personnel are appointed for this function and purchasing officer may assume the following duties:

1. Issue of purchase orders.
2. Maintenance of purchase records.
3. Follow ups on delayed orders.
4. Execution of competitive bidding procedures.
5. Obtaining the quotations from specified sources.

Objectives in Purchasing

The general areas in which purchasing objectives must be established can be named as "Seven Rights of Purchasing." These are – the pharmacy manager should buy:

1. The *right variety* of merchandise.
2. The *right quality* of merchandise to meet the target market's expectations and demands.
3. The *right quantity* of goods at a particular point in time to ensure that the risk of stock-outs are balanced against the costs of tying up funds in excess inventory.
4. At the *right time*, so that the supply of incoming merchandise roughly coincides with customer purchases.
5. From the *right sources* to obtain the most favourable terms possible and develop dependable sources of supply.
6. At the *right price* so that the cost of goods will not be too high to allow for a reasonable gross margin.
7. At the *right cost* to the pharmacy in terms of minimising the expenses associated with purchasing.

Objectives in Inventory Control

There are several objectives of inventory control.

1. Minimization of the inventory investment.
2. Determination of the right level of customer service.
3. Balance of supply and demand.
4. Minimization of procurement costs and carrying costs.
5. Maintenance of an up-to-date inventory control system.

Procedure for Purchasing: The procedure for purchasing the drugs described here assumes that there exist in the hospital, a qualified pharmacist and the purchasing agent. It also assumes that the specifications have been drawn by the pharmacist and all supplies ordered will be received and stored in the pharmacy or store-room controlled by pharmacist. The pharmacist or a person authorised by him, should complete a Purchase Request form for the product desired; which is given on the next page.

Purchase / Repair Request

XYZ Hospital, Pune.

No. 1234

Date ....

- Repair of equipment.
- Purchase

Department Name	Account name charge to	Purchasing Department use only				
Charge Code	Suggested vendor	Terms	Purchase Order Number			
Date Needed	....	Price per unit	Number of units needed	Total Price	Quantity	
					On hand	Used per
Commodity Number	Descriptions – Specifications – Packaging					

Requested by .... Approved by ......

Fig. 7.1: Purchase Request Form

DEPARTMENT OF PHARMACY

X – Y – Z Hospital, Pune.

PURCHASING REQUISITION

Vendor .... Vendor No. .... Purchase Order No. ....

Vendor contact ....

Date placed .... Ordering frequency .... Date prepared ....

Next Ordering Date .... Shipping Date .... Cost Centre No. ....

Prepared By .... Order Taken By ....

No.	Quantity	Unit	Description	Cost each	Extension	Contract Price

Fig. 7.2: Purchase Order Form

The drugs brought from the same vendor can be grouped on a single form. This form contains data regarding description, specifications, packaging, price, quantity needed, inventory balance and anticipated monthly use. This form is also a source of information to the accounting office regarding the cost centre to be charged and the discount whether earned or not after the payment for merchandise. The original of this form is forwarded to the administrative officer. After approval it is forwarded to purchasing agent. A copy is retained by the pharmacist for his record to indicate that goods are in the process of procurement. The purchasing agent after receiving the "Purchase Request" prepares the "Purchase Order" as above. Purchase order must be prepared from the data of Purchase Request Form and it could consist of two or more snap out pages. However a multicopy snap out form is suitable as it provides a copy for:

1. Supplier
2. Accounts department
3. Purchasing number file
4. Department from which purchase is requisitioned
5. Two receiving reports
6. History of the purchase.

The supplier copy is either mailed or hand delivered to his representative. The accounts payable copy is forwarded to the accounting office where it is held until the invoice is received from the supplier and the completed receiving reports from the initiating department. Then only the invoice is processed for payment.

The third copy is retained by the purchasing agent for his number file.

The fourth copy is returned to initiating department. This copy should be matched with "Purchase Request Form" to check for accuracy.

The fifth and sixth copies serve as receiving reports and are sent to receiving department. If the entire order is received, then fifth copy is completed and forwarded to accounting office. If order is received partial and be back ordered, sixth copy is used.

The seventh copy is the history copy and is retained by the purchasing agent for use in ascertaining the rates.

After receiving the merchandise, the pharmacist must record in the purchase records the transaction for every item purchased. This purchase record acts as a source of information for determining rate of use, cost of drugs, its source and such other details. Such purchase record may be maintained by the purchasing agent and made available to the pharmacist when needed.

Sometimes, few drugs which are out of stock may be ordered from the pharmacy. This may happen when pharmacy department handles surgical and laboratory supplies as well as drugs. In such situation the pharmacist should prepare an "out of stock" form in duplicate and one copy should be sent to the ward or laboratory and other copy should be retained in the pharmacy.

X — Y — Z Hospital, Pune Pharmacy Date .... Department .... Name on Original Req. .... We are temporarily out of stock for the following.	
Quantity	**Items**
	❑ Charged ❑ Not charged
When these items are available, your order will be completed PLEASE DO NOT REORDER	

Fig. 7.3: Out of Stock Form

This form for out of stock serves two purposes:

(i) Speedy delivery of merchandise to the ward or laboratory and

(ii) Prevents re-ordering from wards/ laboratory.

Controls on Purchases

A modern and reliable method of controlling the purchases is the computation of inventory turnover.

The Inventory turnover rate represents the average number of times inventory is sold and replaced during a given period. In general, a high turnover rate indicates that merchandise is selling well relative to the average amount of inventory kept in stock. It may be due to small volume purchasing which indicates a failure to take advantage of the maximum quantity discounts. A low turnover rate indicates that merchandise is not moving very quickly relative to average inventory i.e. large purchase of slow moving items and duplication of stock resulting in dead inventory.

A turnover of four to six times a year is considered as satisfactory. Inventory turnover rate is calculated by dividing average inventory by sales. It can be calculated on the basis of retail sales, costs or units. Each of the following formulae will provide identical inventory turnover rates.

$$ITR = \frac{S}{AIRD} = \frac{SC}{AIC} = \frac{U}{AIU}$$

where,
ITR = Inventory turnover rate;
S = Net sales;
SC = Sales at cost (or cost of goods sold);
U = Number of units sold;
AIRD = Average inventory in retail dollars
AIC = Average inventory at cost;
AIU = Average inventory in units.

Turnover rate can be used as a standard for inventory control purposes.

Hospital pharmacist should try to control purchase volume and inventory by the use of 'Economic Order Quantity' (EOQ) and 'Recorder Quantity Level' (RQL). The 'Recorder Quantity Level' is defined as the inventory level that must be reached before additional stock can be ordered.

Economic Order Quantity: One of the best known models for inventory control is the economic order quantity (EOQ). The purpose of this model is to answer two important questions:

1. When should an item be reordered (resulting in procurement cost) ? and
2. What quantity should be ordered (resulting in carrying or holding cost) ? Thus this model can be used to determine how much inventory needs to be carried to meet demand.

Procurement costs include costs of making requisitions, writing orders, receiving and inspecting goods, completing the purchase transaction and maintaining inventory records. These costs are normally fixed, regardless of the size of the order.

Carrying costs include such items as interest, insurance, taxes, deterioration, spoilage, obsolescence, handling and warehousing. Because a significant portion of pharmacy's working capital is tied up in inventory, a small reduction in inventory investment may result in a significant increase in working capital and reduce the amount of money needed to borrow. Even if a pharmacy does not borrow to finance its inventory, it would be advantageous to reduce inventory levels since the money can be invested elsewhere. The formula for calculating EOQ is:

$$EOQ = \sqrt{\frac{2 \times D \times PC}{ICC \times UC}}$$

where, D = Annual demand (in units)

PC = Procurement cost (cost to place one order)

ICC = Inventory carrying cost (as % of unit cost)

and UC = Unit costs

The EOQ model is based on following assumptions:

1. The annual usage of particular item of inventory is known.
2. The rate of usage of inventory does not vary over time and
3. Orders placed to replenish the inventory are received at exactly the point in time when inventory is zero.

These assumptions greatly reduce the usefulness of EOQ formula. The useful feature of this model is its determination of a basic optimal reorder quantity that the pharmacy manager may adjust according to his personal knowledge of demand fluctuations, delivery delays etc.

Purchase Timing (Reorder Point)

The reordering time must closely coincide with the consumer demand and minimise the mount of inventory investment. It means to establish stock levels at which new orders must be placed. The stock levels are called reorder points. Determining reorder points depends on the length of order lead time, usage rate and the amount of safety stock lo be kept on the hand.

Order lead time is the time span from the date when an order is placed to the date the merchandise is received, priced and put on the selling floor. Usage rate means average sales per day in units of merchandise. Safety stock is the amount of extra inventory kept on hand to protect against running out of stock owing to unexpected demand and delays in delivery.

The formula for when to reorder is:

Reorder point = (Usage rate × Lead time) + Safety stock

Ideally, orders should be placed at precise point in time at which sales during the order lead time will just have depleted all of the inventory on hand, so that no safety stock is needed.

Decision on What to Control (ABC Analysis)

Some items in the inventory need to be controlled more than others. Some cost more and therefore represent a greater financial investment. Some are dated and have only a relatively short shelf life. Because of this, inventory can be labelled as being A, B or C merchandise. This gives recognition to the varying importance of different types of pharmacy inventory. Consequently, classifying merchandise (items) into A, B and C items allows the pharmacy manager to better identify and control items of greater importance.

As shown in Fig. 7.4 a relatively small percentage of total merchandise represents a very large percentage of investment in inventory.

For example, approximately 20% of the inventory items should receive much greater attention than the remaining 80% since they may account for 90% or more of inventory investment. Loss of control over a few of these items is considerably more serious than loss of control over a large number of other items.

Merchandise 'A' would be considered the most important to control. This includes prescription department inventory, high cost front end merchandise and those considered essential in a full-line pharmacy (e.g. over the counter drugs [OTCs] such as cough syrup, aspirin and antacids). Prescription department inventory is generally most important since it is expensive, essential to store operations and has a limited shelf life. However, high cost front end items and those necessary to maintain the image of the store must be carefully controlled. Accordingly, these 'A' items should be the primary focus of the pharmacy manager's efforts to control inventory.

'C' items on the other hand are the least important to control. These are less expensive items which account for a small investment in inventory and are not especially bulky so as to consume disproportionate amount of shelf space. 'B' items are somewhere in the middle and their control depends on the actual cost of inventory control.

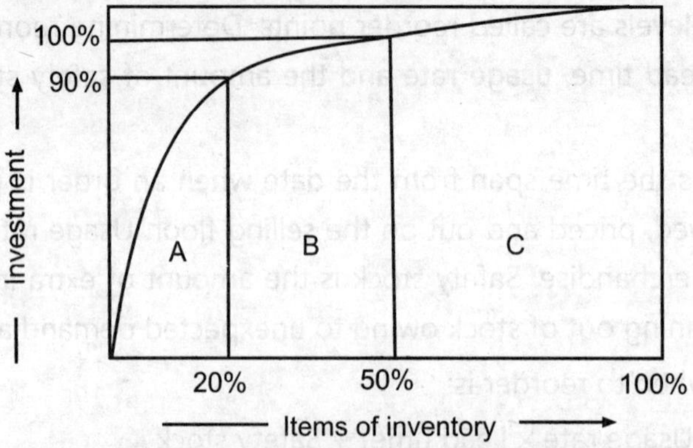

Fig. 7.4: Economic Order Quantity

Testing of Raw Materials

This is the most important stage in the manufacture of pharmaceutical products. To get a high quality product one has to use the best quality of raw materials. Hence, testing of raw materials is of great significance in quality control.

The standards of purity and strength stated in the monograph of the pharmacopoeia apply to articles which are intended for medicinal use only but not necessarily to articles which may be sold under the same name for other purposes.

All statements in the monographs given under the heading 'standards' constitute the standards for the official substances and a substance is not of pharmacopoeial quality unless it complies with all the requirements stated under 'standards'.

Monographs may also include information on chemical formula, molecular weight, category, doses, description and statements under the heading solubility.

The requirements given in the monograph are not framed to provide against all possible impurities. The tests have been framed to fix the limits of impurities which can be tolerated to a given extent.

Expression of Standards

Where the standards for a substance/anhydrous substance described in a monograph is expressed in terms of the chemical formula for that substance/ anhydrous substance and an upper limit is not stated, the upper limit is not more than the equivalent of 100.5 percent.

When a standard is required to be calculated with reference to different conditions of substance, different parameters are determined by methods described in the monograph such as:

Condition of the substance	Parameter to be determined
Dried substance	Loss on drying (LOD)
Anhydrous substance	Content of water
Solvent free substance	Content of solvent

Limits and Tolerances

When limits of content are given in a monograph, they are determined by the method prescribed therein. When limits are expressed in numbers it includes both upper and lower limit numericals and intermediate values.

Usual Strength: The usual strength of the drug of marketed preparation is given in the monograph.

Expression of Strength: With one of the following four different terms, the strength is expressed:

(i) Percent W/W: Number of grams of active substance in 100 grams of product.

(ii) Percent W/V: Number of grams of active substance in 100 millilitres of product.

(iii) Percent V/V: Number of millilitres of active substance in 100 millilitres of product.

(iv) Percent V/W: Number of millilitres of active substance in 100 grams of product.

When the strength of solution is expressed as:

(i) Parts by weight: Weight (grams) of solid in volume (millilitres) of final solution.

(ii) Parts by volume: Volume (millilitres) of a liquid in volume (millilitres) of the final solution.

(iii) Parts by weight: Weight (grams) of gas in weight (grams) of the final solution.

Limits of Impurities: In certain substances the limits of impurities are given approximately in terms - parts per million by weight (ppm) or percentage.

Odour and taste: Whenever a substance is described in the monograph as "odourless", immediately after opening the package, examine not more than 25 g of the sample. If any odour, then transfer the sample rapidly to an open container and re-examine after 15 minutes.

If still there is odour, the sample does not comply with the description 'odourless'.

The tests of odour and taste are descriptive only and not regarded as standards of purity for a particular lot.

Solubility: It is also not a standard or test for purity of a substance except where a quantitative solubility test is given under standards, the substance should comply with this requirement.

The solubility of a substance is indicated by a descriptive term and is intended to apply at ambient temperature.

Descriptive Term	Approximate Quantity of Solvent for 1 Part of Solute
Very soluble	Less than 1 part
Freely soluble	From 1 to 10 parts
Soluble	From 10 to 30 parts
Sparingly soluble	From 30 to 100
Slightly soluble	From 100 to 1000 parts
Very slightly soluble	From 1000 to 10,000 parts
Insoluble	More than 10,000 parts

Tests and Assays

Methods are described under the monograph for each drug.

Apparatus: Specifications for apparatus are given merely as recommendations. Where volumetric flasks or exact measuring or weighing devices are specified, then that specific or other equipments of equivalent accuracy can be used.

Solutions of higher or lower concentrations should be prepared with the solvent specified in the procedure in order to obtain these in the working range of the instrument being used.

Water-bath: Water-bath means a bath of boiling water, unless water at some other temperature is indicated.

Desiccator: A tightly closed container of suitable size that maintains an atmosphere of low moisture content. Silica gel or phosphorus pentoxide is usually used as desiccant.

Vacuum Desiccator: Maintains the low moisture atmosphere at a reduced pressure of ≯20 Torr.

Percentage of Alcohol: The term 'Alcohol content' refers to percentage by volume of C_2H_5OH at 15.56°C. Only when 'C_2H_5OH' is mentioned absolute (100%) strength is intended.

Reagents and Solutions: The quality of the reagents and solutions used in tests and assays greatly affects the results. These should be prepared and used as defined in the appendices of I.P.

The abbreviation 'Sp' is employed for reagents for the limit tests for heavy metals and lead.

Reference Substances and Standard preparations: These are the antibiotic and other substances which are authentic specimens used as comparison standards in some of the tests and assays pharmacopoeia. The word 'I.P. reference substance' is abbreviated to RS.

Solvents: Where the name of the solvent is not stated, water is used for preparation solution. When water is specified, purified water is to be used. Distilled water indicates purified water of a prepared by distillation. The term 'alcohol' means 95% v/v ethanol and 'ethyl alcohol' means absolute alcohol of I.P. standard.

Procedures: Assay and test procedures are provided for determining compliance with the pharmacopoeial standards. The methods are given in I.P. but the analyst may use alternative methods such as automated procedures and micro-analysis, provided the results obtained are of equivalent accuracy.

Assay: The quantity to be taken is indicated approximately but quantity actually used must be accurately weighed. It should not be deviated by more than 10% from that stated.

Test: The quantity to be taken is indicated and must be taken exactly.

Blank determination: Same procedure is to be followed except the sample.

Indicator: Approximately 0.1 ml or 3 drops should be used, unless otherwise directed.

Negligible: It means not more than 0.5 mg.

Pressure: It is indicated in mm of Hg or Torr.

Temperature: Indicated in Celsius scale and all measurements are made at 25°C unless otherwise specified.

Time Limit: 5 minutes should be allowed for the reaction to take pace, unless otherwise specified.

Biological/Microbiological Tests and Assays

The methods are described in the appendices of I.P.

The biological assay methods are provided for two purposes viz. (i) To ascertain purity, and (ii) To determine total activity of the drug.

Packaging Storage and Labelling

Container is the device that holds the product. The material of container should not interact with its contents so as to change its strength, quality or purity.

Immediate Container: One which is in direct contact with the contents.

Light Resistant Container: One which protects the contents from light because of the specific properties of the material of container. The clear or colourless container may be made light resistant by means of an opaque covering.

Well-closed Container: The container which protects the contents from extraneous solids and from loss of contents during handling, shipment, storage and distribution.

Tightly Closed Container: A container which protects the contents from contamination by extraneous solids, liquids or vapours and from loss by effervescence, deliquescence or evaporation under normal conditions of handling, shipment, storage and distribution. It must be capable of being tightly reclosed after use.

Hermetically Sealed Container: It is the container which is impervious to air or any other gas under normal conditions of handling, shipment, storage an distribution.

Single dose container - for parenterals

Multidose container - for parenterals

Storage: Following descriptive terms are used for directions of storage.

(a) Cold: Temperature between 2° to 8°C.

(b) Cool: Temperature between 8° to 25°C.

(c) Room temperature.

(d) Warm: Temperature between 30°-40°C.

(e) Excessive heat: Temperature above 40°C.

Labelling: Labelling of drugs is governed by the rules made under the Drugs and Cosmetics Act, 1940.

Weights and Measures: The metric system is to be followed.

QUESTIONS

1. Explain the role of pharmacist in purchasing of drugs.
2. What is the role of purchasing officer in purchasing?
3. Give the objectives of "Purchasing" and "Inventory control."
4. Describe the procedure for purchasing of drugs.
5. Write short notes on:
   (i) Inventory turnover rate
   (ii) EOQ
   (iii) Reorder point (RO)
   (iv) ABC - analysis
6. Give the format for (i) Purchase request form, and (ii) 'Out of stock' form.
7. Name the various tests prescribed in I.P. for testing a drug.
8. In which different forms, the strength is expressed?
9. Write a note on "containers for packaging" as per I.P.

***

8

HOSPITAL INSTRUMENTS AND HEALTH ACCESSORIES

No surgeon can be successful without the use of surgical instruments. However the expansion of modern technology has provided us with alternatives to the basic instruments. The diagnostic tools are more important to the surgeon as his surgical instruments. Accurate diagnosis is essential for an appropriate and effective treatment. Without the use of fibrelight instruments we would not be able to visualise directly the duodenum, bile ducts, colon or even joints. Ultrasound and CT scan have provided us a safe non-invasive tool of adequate accuracy. Almost any hollow body cavity can be directly visualised with the use of simple apparatus. The major blood vessels or heart can be intubated for sampling, monitoring or transfusion. Now-a-days human organs are being replaced with artificial ones.

For study purposes, hospital instruments can be classified into three categories:

I. Diagnostic instruments,

II. Therapeutic instruments, and

III. Operative instruments.

(I) DIAGNOSTIC INSTRUMENTS

The instruments used for diagnostic purpose are:

(A) Optical Instruments

(i) **Laryngoscope and Pharyngoscope:** These are instruments designed for direct examination of larynx and it is most commonly used by anaesthetists for intubation.

(ii) **Bronchoscope:** It is used for direct visualisation of the trachea and bronchial tree. It is used for diagnostic as well as therapeutic purposes.

(iii) **Mediastinoscope:** It is used for examination and biopsy of superior mediastinal lymph nodes which frequently involves in bronchial carcinoma.

(iv) **Gastrointestional endoscopy:**

Oesophagoscope: It is used for examination of oesophagus.

The rigid oesophagoscope of Negus or Chevalier-Jackson pattern is a hollow tube about 45 cm long and 16-20 mm in diameter. The instrument is calibrated in centimeters from the distal end and on its anterior side. To facilitate the insertion, a rigid handle at the right angle to its long axis is provided. Modern instruments use fibre optic illumination.

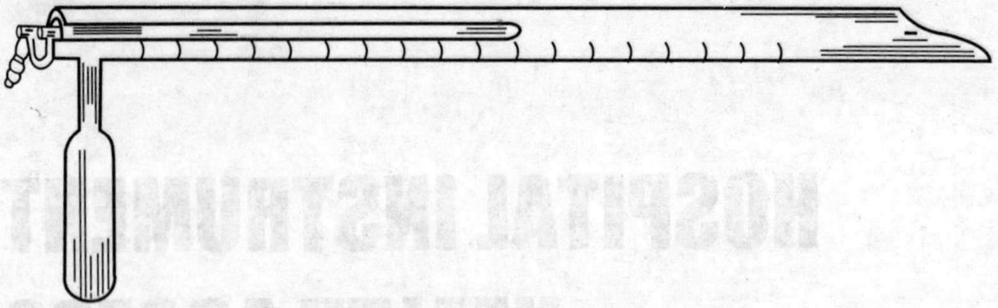

Fig. 8.1: Negus Oesophagoscope

(v) Choledochoscope: Choledochoscopy is the technique of visualisation of the common and hepatic bile ducts through choledochotomy. It improves diagnostic accuracy of bile duct exploration. The rigid choledochoscope is an L-shaped instrument with lighting, viewing and irrigating systems. Saline is used for irrigation. The instrument is sterilised in ethylene oxide gas. The standard choledochotomy incision allows the introduction of the instrument having 5 × 3 mm diameter.

The instrument is first inserted towards the ampulla and then advanced further under direct vision until the sphincter of a common bile duct is seen. The instrument is then withdrawn, rotated by 180° and reinserted through choledochotomy to visualise the hepatic ducts.

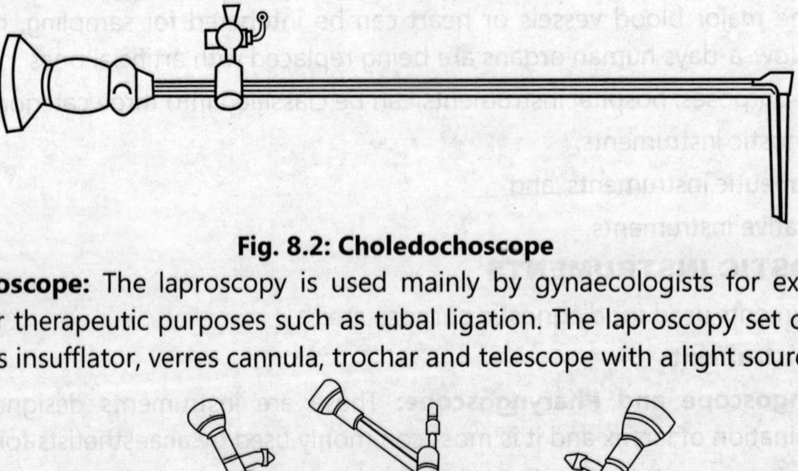

Fig. 8.2: Choledochoscope

(vi) Laproscope: The laproscopy is used mainly by gynaecologists for examination of pelvis and for therapeutic purposes such as tubal ligation. The laproscopy set consists of an automatic gas insufflator, verres cannula, trochar and telescope with a light source.

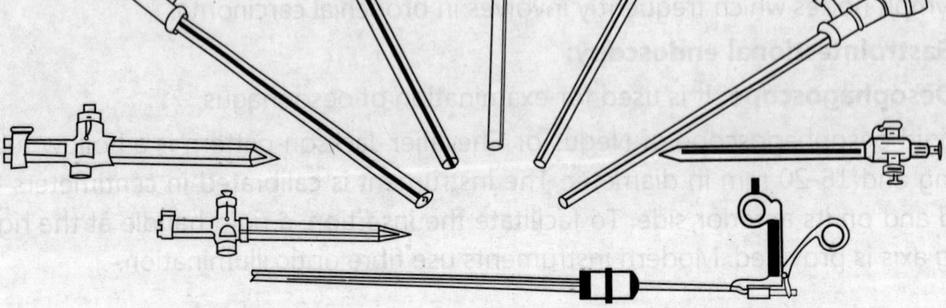

Fig. 8.3: A Range of Olympus Laproscope and Accessories

(vii) Arthroscope: It is used for endoscopic examination of joints. It has an advantage over exploratory arthrotomy as it lowers risk of infection and morbidity. The knee joint is most accessible for this type of examination. Knee arthroscopy is indicated in injuries and chondromalacia patellae, osteochondritis dissecans and arthritis.

It is a rigid instrument consisting of steel sheath, trochars and telescopes. The sheath is attached to an irrigating system and is 5 mm in diameter. If biopsy forceps are used, the standard 4 mm telescope is replaced with 2.7 mm telescope to accommodate both within the sheath.

(viii) Urological endoscopy: Ureteroscope is the recent addition in the field of urology. It is less invasive than percutaneous nephroscopy and it is useful in a large number of patients to visualise the renal pelvis.

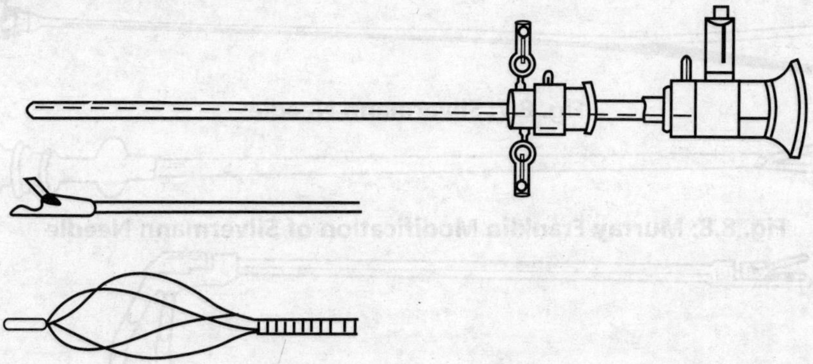

Fig. 8.4: Ureteroscope

(B) CT Scan

Computerised axial tomography provides information about tissue density in a thin section of tissue. This technique was developed in 1972 by N. Hounsfield. The idea was based on the assumption that measurement of X-rays passing through the body could provide information on all tissues in the path of an X-ray beam. When the beam is multidirectional and data obtained is computed and presented in such a form to produce a three-dimensional picture.

(C) Biopsies

Biopsy is defined as examination of living tissue removed from the body.

The most direct way of taking a biopsy is to cut away a piece of tissue with a scalpel under direct vision. It is a formal operation often requiring anaesthesia and incision results in a scar.

1. Curette: The curette is a scoop-like instrument used to scrap off material or tissue for biopsy.

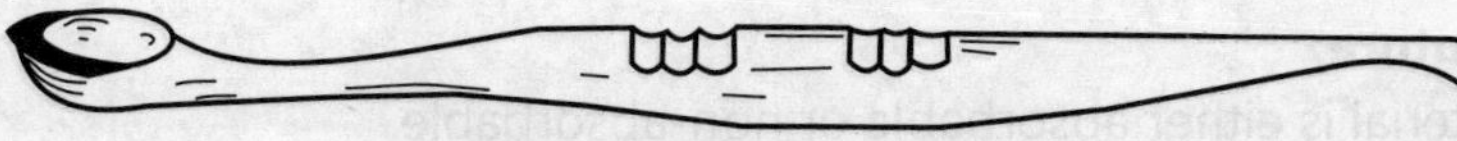

Fig. 8.5: Volkmann Scoop

2. Needle biopsy: It is the most frequently used technique of biopsy due to its simplicity and speed. The main advantage of this technique is that it can be performed under local anaesthesia with minimum facilities and minimum trauma.

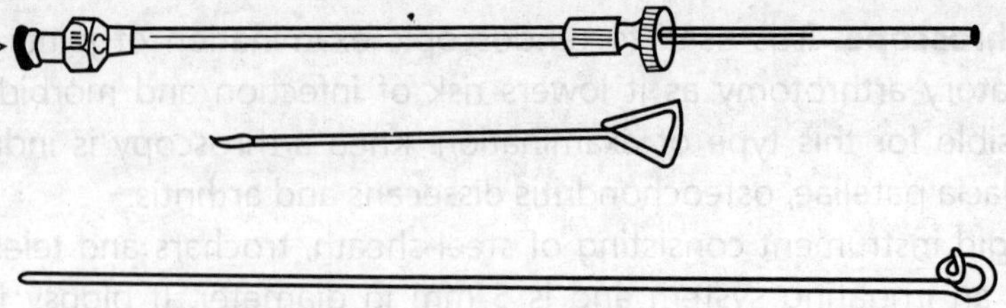

Fig. 8.6: Menghini Needle

3. **Biopsy Punch Forceps:** These are used to remove a piece of tissue by occlusion of two cupped jaws. These are suitable for mucosal biopsies.

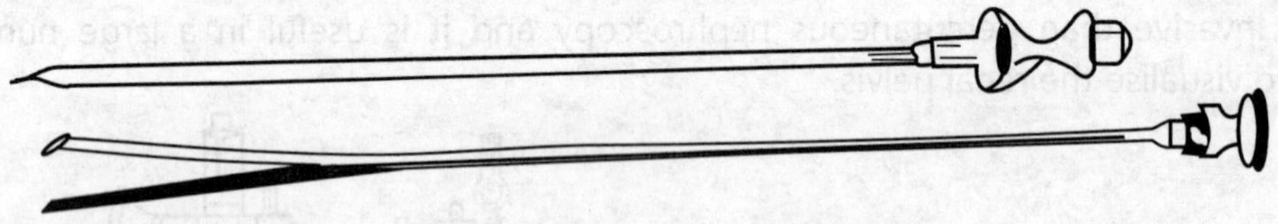

Fig. 8.7: Silvermann Needle

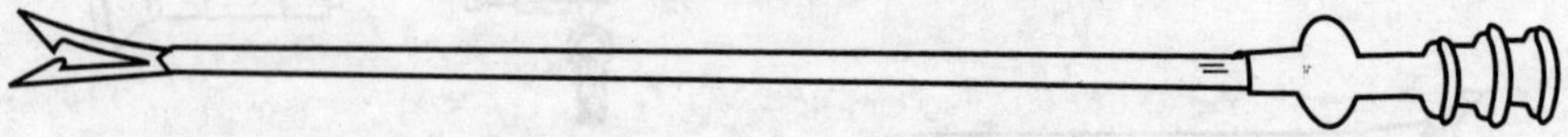

Fig. 8.8: Murray Franklin Modification of Silvermann Needle

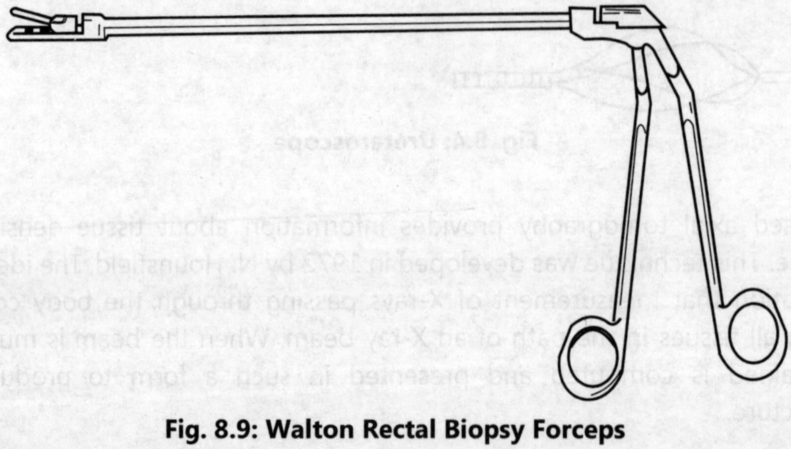

Fig. 8.9: Walton Rectal Biopsy Forceps

(II) THERAPEUTIC INSTRUMENTS

(a) Equipments for Sterilization

(i) Autoclave

(ii) Hot air oven

(iii) Chemical sterilizer

(b) Surgical Suture

Suture material is either absorbable or non-absorbable.

1. **Catgut:** It is an absorbable material. It is made from the strips of sheep gut submucosa which is subjected to mechanical cleaning so that the final product consists of pure collagen. The ribbons are then twisted together and chromed, if desired, dried under tension and polished. It is sterilized by ethylene oxide or gamma radiation.

2. Silk: It is non-absorbable suture produced from the silkworm larva thread. It is stronger than catgut and can be boiled or autoclaved. Since it absorbs fluid, it is treated with silicone or wax to render it non-permeable.

3. Cotton: It is rarely used and has poor tensile strength.

4. Linen: It is made from twisted staple flax fibres. It is stronger than cotton. It produces vigorous tissue reaction. It is cheap and easy for handling.

5. Nylon: It is a synthetic polyamide. Although it is strong, it has poor knot tying qualities and it looses its strength after six months in tissues. It is also brittle.

Newer synthetic materials are made of polyesters, polyethylenes or polypropylene.

(c) Surgical Gloves

It is an essential barrier between patient and surgeon, serving to protect both from infection. The early surgical gloves were made of thick valcanised rubber. They were reusable and after use were washed, repaired and sterilized. Now-a-days gloves are made from latex rubber. In order to produce an outer textured and inner smooth surface, the gloves are manufactured inside out. To prevent the dry surface of gloves sticking together they must be dusted with powder. Gloves are supplied with a sachet of powders. Starch powder and talc is generally used.

(d) Equipments for Drains and Splints

1. Gastric and Intestinal Tubes: These tubes can be passed into the stomach or even beyond for decompression, sampling or delivery of drugs or food. These are also used for stomach washouts.

E.g.

1. Gastric lavage tube
2. Ryle's gastroduodenal tube
3. Miller-Abbott tube.

2. Abdominal and Chest Drains: The drains are used to prevent fluid collection within the abdominal cavity; drainage of fluid from pleural cavity and to avoid the obliteration of cavities.

Drains used following thoroacic surgery are simply plastic or rubber tubes with or without side holes in the intrapleural portion of the drain.

3. Urological Catheters: These are used to decompress or splint any part of urinary system.

The Foley catheter is a plastic two-lumen tube with an integral inflatable balloon. Modern urethral catheters are made of materials which are least irritant to urethra. Silastic is the least irritant but it is soft and expensive. This material is particularly suitable for long-term, catheterization. Latex coated with polysiloxane elastomer is superior to latex, but these catheters are thicker with smaller lumen. Also these are collapsible under suction and therefore less suitable where bladder washout is required. This problem can be avoided by using PVC catheters with a latex balloon. The advantages of using PVC are:

1. Its firmness avoids the need for catheter introducer.
2. Its thermoplasticity softens the catheter at body temperature.
3. The aspiration does not result in luminal collapse.

The choice of catheter tip is important. It can be straight or curved. The curved catheters are called coude and are specifically designed to pass the prostatic urethra distorted by prostatic enlargement.

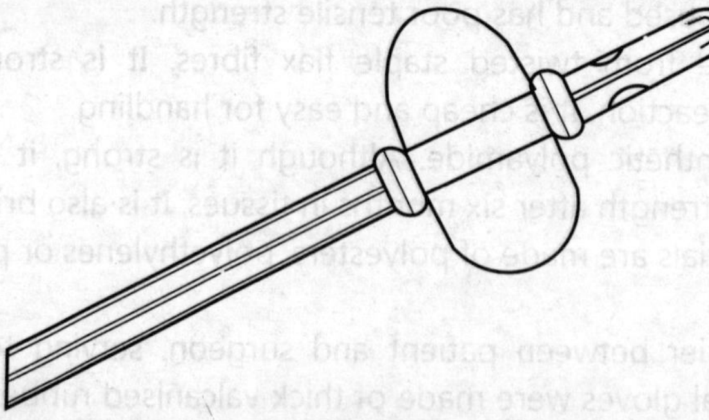

Fig. 8.10: Foley Balloon Catheter

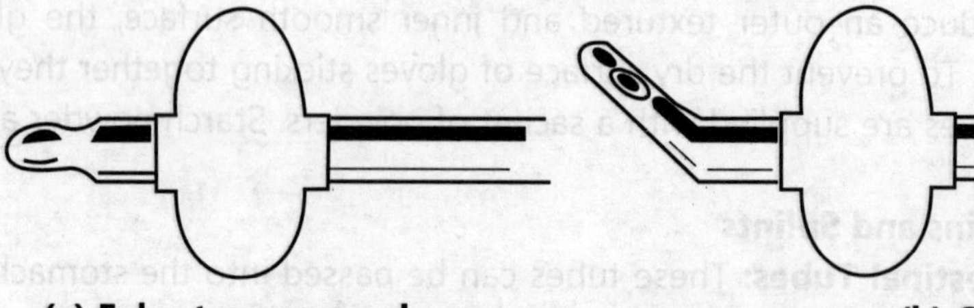

(a) Foley two opposed eyes **(b) Coude**

Fig. 8.11: Urethral Catheter tips

4. Endotracheal Tubes and Tracheostomy Tube: These tubes are used for relief of upper respiratory obstruction. These are also used for ventilation of lungs and for anaesthesia purposes. The tubes are used for prolonged ventilation in major head and neck surgery, in patients with deficient swallowing reflexes and in cases of laryngitis and epiglotitis.

(e) Laser

It means 'light amplification by stimulated emission of radiation'.

Its power is derived from a beam of light of uniform wavelength which on contact with an absorptive surface liberates heat. Tissues exposed to this light beam coagulate or are evaporated.

The effect of the laser beam on tissues depends on its spectrum, energy and tissue absorption. Currently, there are three types of lasers used in surgery, namely CO_2, argon and neodymium YAG.

CO_2 laser uses a mixture of CO_2 and nitrogen. The active medium is CO_2 and nitrogen acts to transfer energy from the pump to CO_2 molecules.

Argon laser uses argon gas as the active medium and an electric current as a pump.

Neodymium - yttrium - aluminium - garnet (YAG) laser is a solid state laser which uses a krypton or xenon lamp as a pump.

Laser coagulates small vessels as it cuts. It is used 'mainly for treatment of superficial skin lesions and in the gastrointestinal tract for bleeding and treatment of vascular lesions.

(f) Lithotripsy

It is the technique used to disintegrate urinary stone by a laser beam.

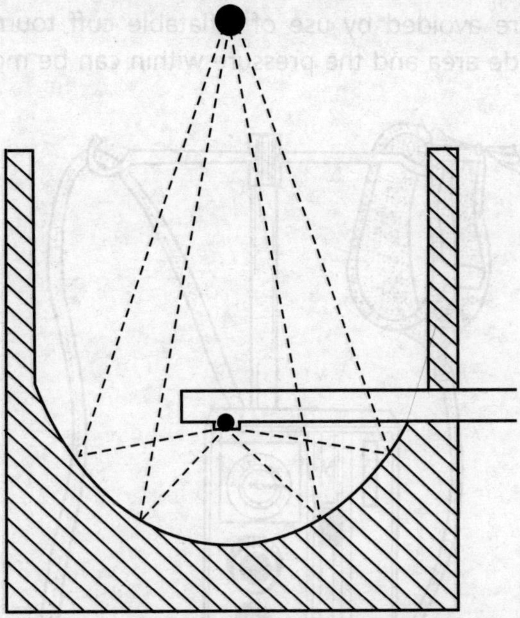

Fig. 8.12: Shock Wave Generator

The basic principle of shock wave lithotripsy is the generation of shock waves which are directed to the stone by means of two image intensifier cameras. The shock waves are produced by an underwater spark discharge between two electrodes situated in an ellipsoidal reflector. They are generated in a medium of water. The ellipsoidal reflector serves to reflect the waves in such a manner that they are concentrated in small area. The waves are then coupled to the medium and reflected to a focal point.

The Dornier lithotripter is composed of a shock wave generator, coupling tub and frame, location system and patient positioning system. The shock waves are produced in an ellipsoidal reflector between two electrodes immersed in water. The coupling medium is specially treated water, contained in a stainless steel tub.

The location system consists of two X-ray tubes located in such a way that their beams intersect in the second focus of the reflection. The two X-ray cameras are placed exactly in the line of each X-ray beam and the picture is displayed on a monitor. The patient positioning allows the adjustment of kidney stone into the focal point of shock wave reflection.

This technique of disintegrating the urinary stone is non-invasive and does not cause any organ damage.

(g) Tourniquet

The simple tourniquet is an elastic band which is in daily use in all hospitals. It is used for venepuncture or insertion of peripheral venous cannulae. The main use of tourniquet is for controlling haemorrhage. The two main disadvantages of these tourniquets are:

(i) Pressure exerted is very localised.

(ii) Inaccurate pressure is exerted.

These disadvantages are avoided by use of inflatable cuff tourniquet. This tourniquet exerts a pressure over a wide area and the pressure within can be monitored and altered at will.

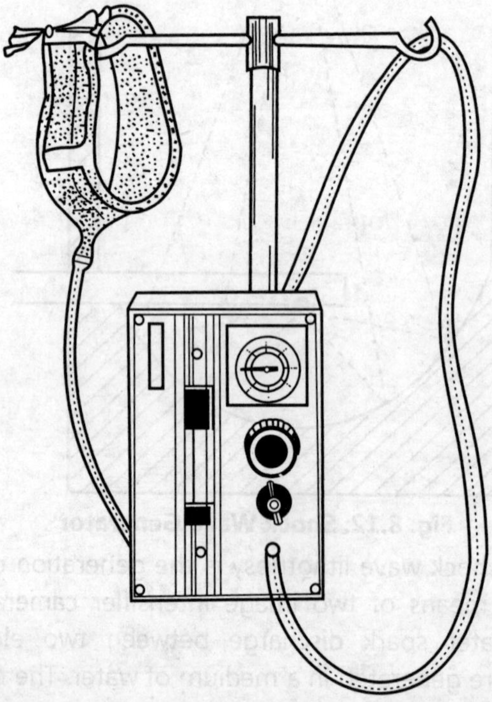

Fig. 8.13: Kidde Standard Pneumatic Tourniquet

It is used mainly in limb surgery where complete stoppage of blood for a prolonged period of time is required. It should be used with care. Inadequate pressure may result in venous congestion and oedema. It should be used with regular release to prevent irreversible ischaemia.

(III) OPERATIVE INSTRUMENTS (SURGICAL INSTRUMENTS)

The following instruments are used at the time of the general surgery.

1. Scalpel: The scalpel is a small knife used in surgical operations. It is invariably used for incision and dissection. It is made up of metal blade with a handle of bone or wood to the complete steel instrument.

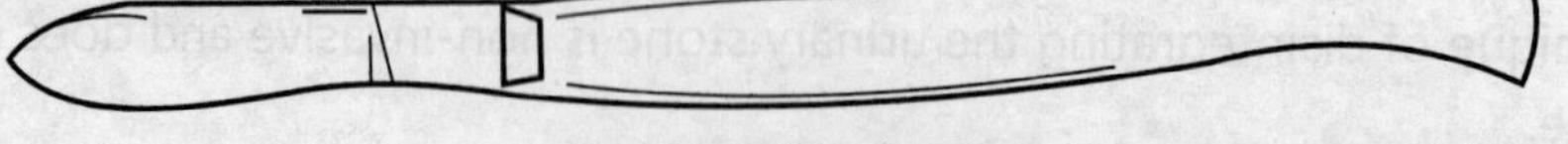

Fig. 8.14: Scalpel

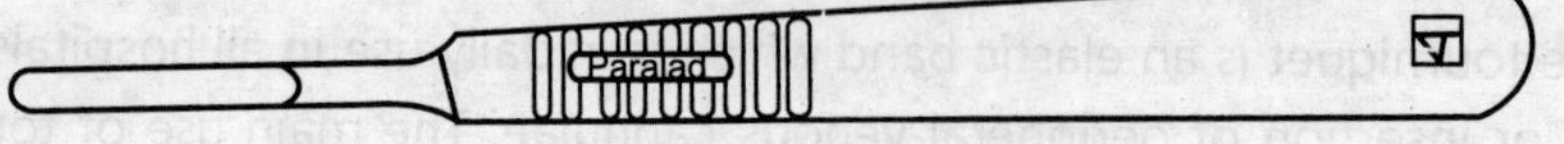

Fig. 8.15: Scalpel Handle

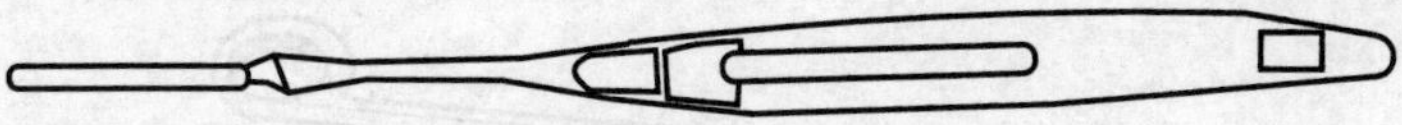

Fig. 8.16: Scalpel handle

2. **Scissors:** Most surgical scissors are dissecting scissors and have chamfered ends. Cutting takes place at the moving point of contact between the edges of two blades. The choice of surgical scissors is vast. They can be long or short, strong or fine, blunt or sharp pointed, straight or curved either on the flat side or on the edge. More expensive scissors have tungsten edges which are sharp, tough and long lasting. The short scissors are used for surface cuttings whereas long scissors are used for deep dissection such as thoracic and pelvic surgery.

The curved scissors are more popular for dissection because, with the convexity of blades pointing away from the surgeon, structures being cut on both the sides of the tip are visible.

Mayo's Scissors: It is most popular among short scissors. Both straight or curved scissors are available for fine surgical dissection.

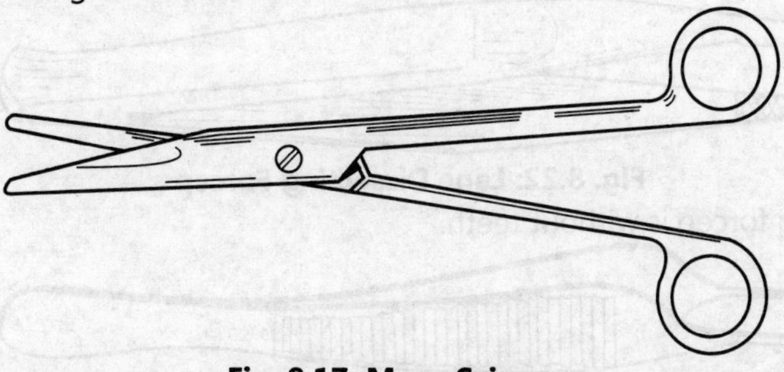

Fig. 8.17: Mayo Scissor

McIndoe Scissors: This scissor is of intermediate length 7 inch long and curved.

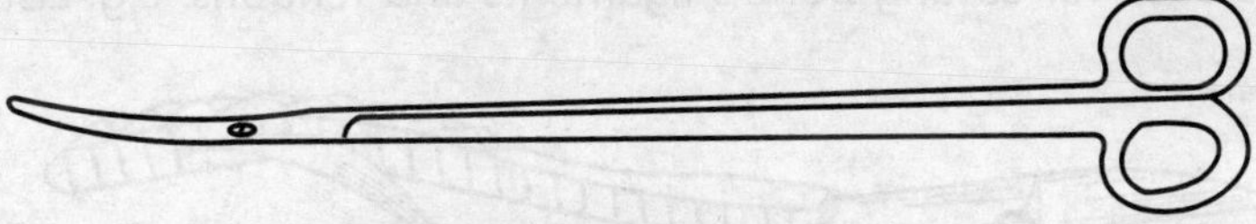

Fig. 8.18: McIndoe Scissor

Long Scissors

(a) Nelson Scissors: It has a shorter and thinner blade. It is basically designed for thoracic surgery.

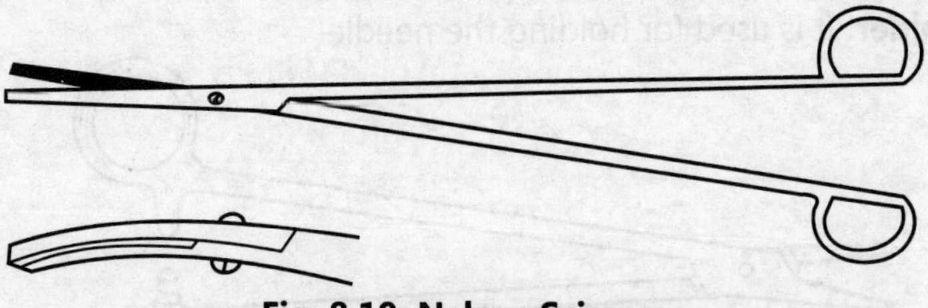

Fig. 8.19: Nelson Scissors

In case of pelvic surgery, the tough ligaments and pedicles need to be cut and this requires strong scissors with blunt edges. The examples of such scissors are Lloyd Davis rectal scissors, and Abel scissors.

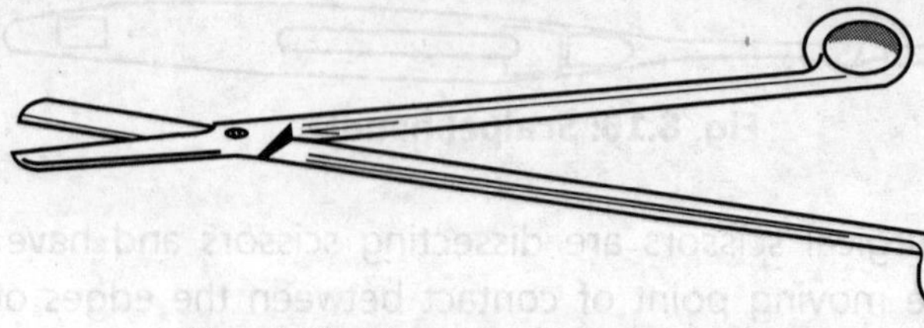

Fig. 8.20: Lloyd Davis Rectal Scissor

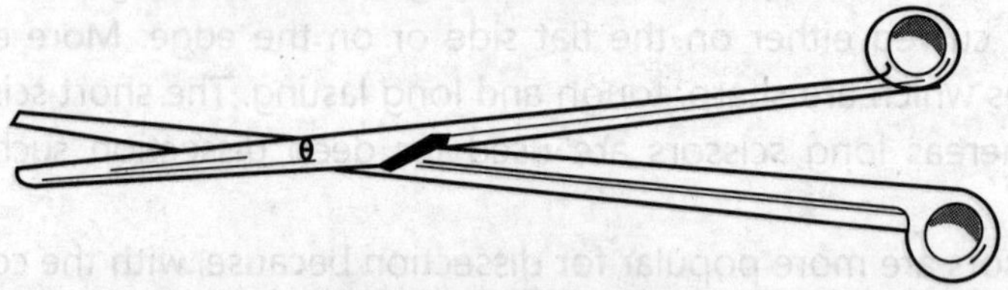

Fig. 8.21: Abel Scissor

3. **Dissecting Forceps with Teeth:** It is used for holding skin, muscle etc. during suturing e.g. Lane's dissecting forceps.

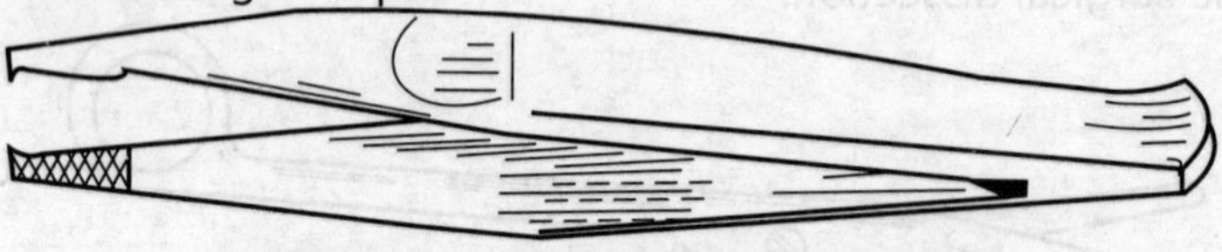

Fig. 8.22: Lane Dissecting Forcep

Adson dissecting forcep is without teeth.

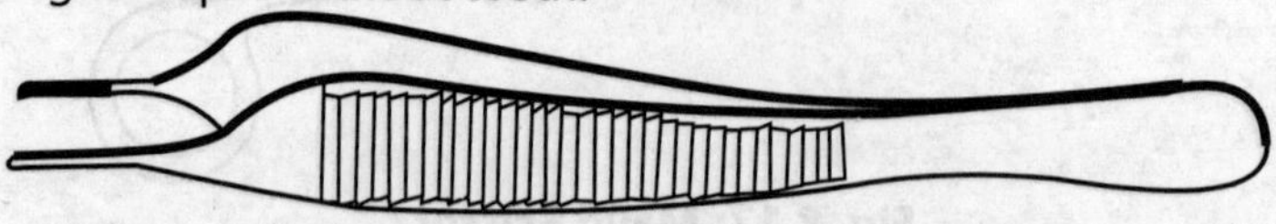

Fig. 8.23: Adson Dissecting Forcep

4. **Cutter:** It is used for cutting bone's ligaments and tendons. e.g. *Liston* bone cutting forceps.

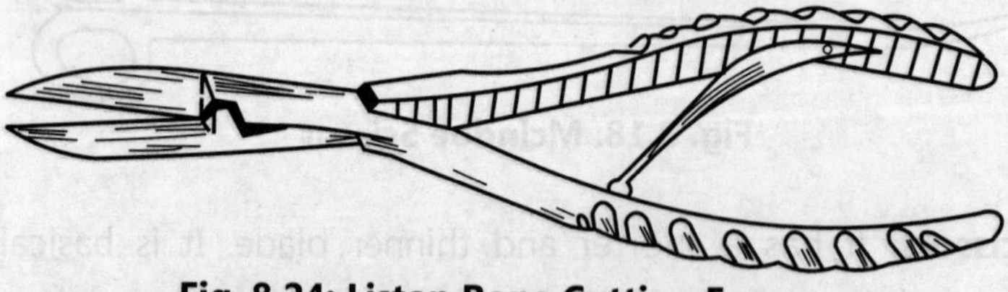

Fig. 8.24: Liston Bone Cutting Forcep

5. **Needle Holder:** It is used for holding the needle.

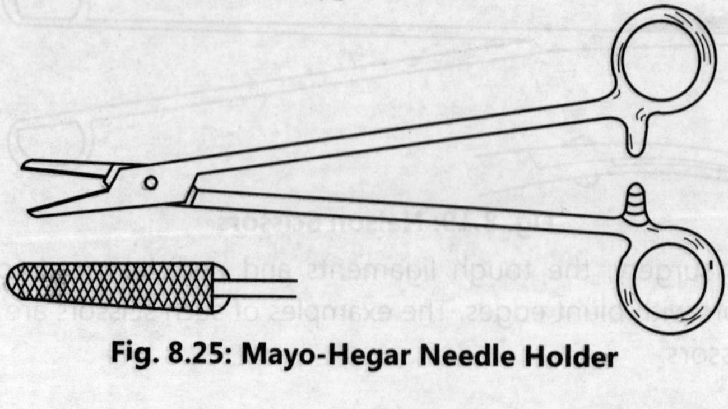

Fig. 8.25: Mayo-Hegar Needle Holder

6. Kocher's Artery Forceps: It is used to pick up retracting blood vessels in the peritoneum and fibrous tissue.

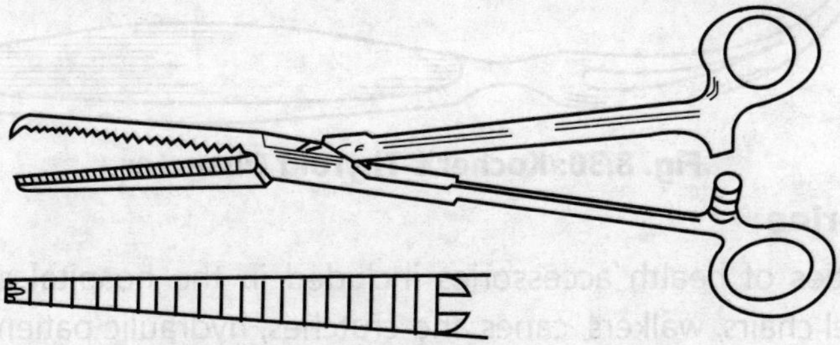

Fig. 8.26: Kocher's Artery Forcep

7. Allis Tissue Forceps: Because of the special structure of teeth of the forceps, it is useful for holding the bowel at the time of anastomosis.

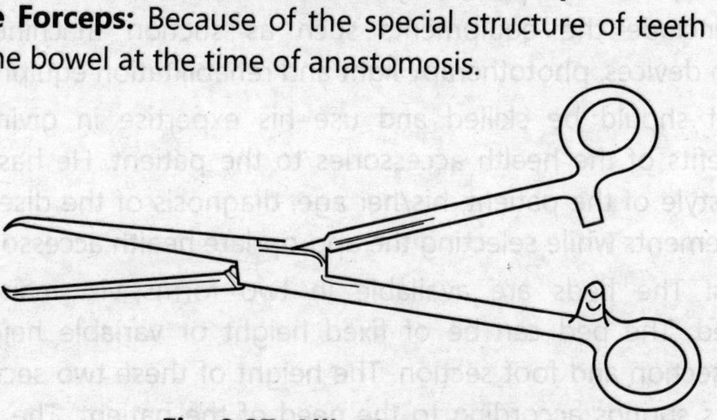

Fig. 8.27: Allis Tissue Forcep

8. Lane's Tissue Forceps: It is used for holding tissues. The holes in the blade allow bulging of tissue, thereby giving a better grip and causing minimum damage to the tissue.

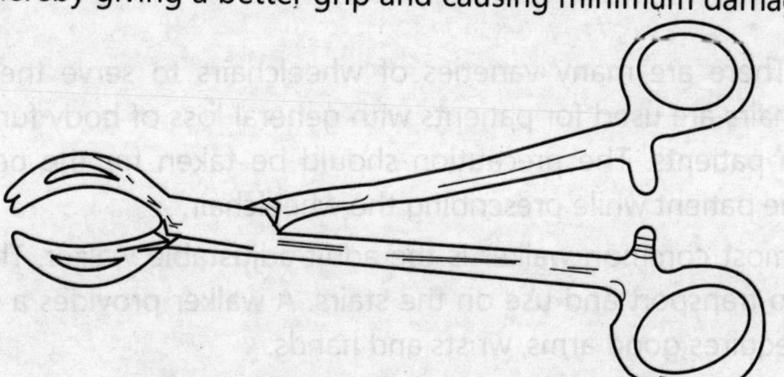

Fig. 8.28: Lane's Tissue Forcep

9. Kocher's Intestinal Clamp: It is used to hold the intestine.

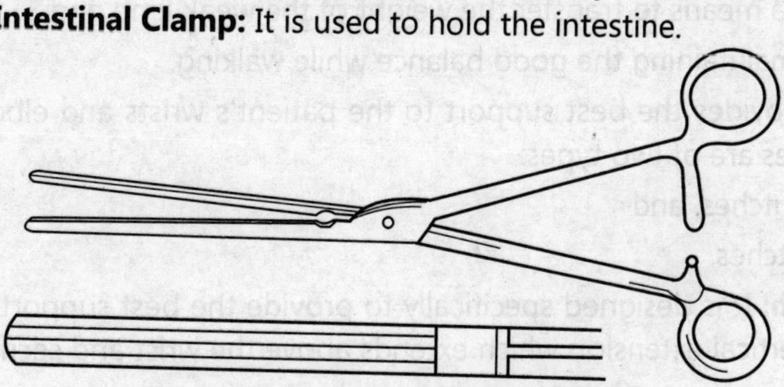

Fig. 8.29: Kocher's Intestinal Clamp

10. Kochce's Thyroid Dissector: It is used for dissecting thyroid during its operation.

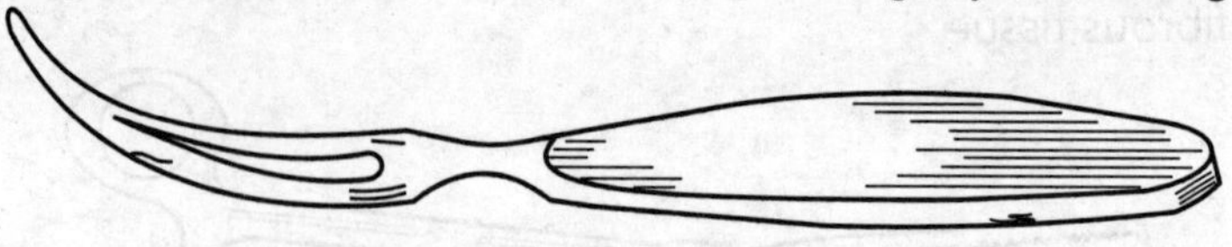

Fig. 8.30: Kocher's Thyroid Dissector

Health Accessories

The wide varieties of health accessories included in the hospital are surgical supplies, hospital beds, wheel chairs, walkers, canes and crutches, hydraulic patient lifters, urology and incontinence supplies, ostomy appliances, orthopaedic braces and elastic supports. Many pharmacies also include the equipments such as suction machines, oxygen therapy equipment, traction devices, phototherapy light and rehabilitation equipment.

The pharmacist should be skilled and use his expertise in giving help and advice regarding the benefits of the health accessories to the patient. He has to consider certain factors such as lifestyle of the patient, his/her age, diagnosis of the disease and patient and equipment measurements while selecting the appropriate health accessory.

Hospital Beds: The beds are available in two forms viz. manually opeıated and electrically operated. The bed can be of fixed height or variable height. Beds have two sections viz. head section and foot section. The height of these two sections of the bed can be adjusted with its springs according to the need of the patient. The bed side safety rails have clamps which can be attached to the steel parts of the spring. The typical overhead trapeze bar can also be used by the patient that helps in sitting up and getting into and out of the bed.

Wheelchairs: There are many varieties of wheelchairs to serve the patient's different needs. The wheelchairs are used for patients with general loss of body functions especially in the aged or infirm patients. The precaution should be taken for the perfect fitting of the accessory to suit the patient while prescribing the wheelchair.

Walkers: The most common walker is the adult adjustable walker. The folding walker is more convenient to transport and use on the stairs. A walker provides a steadier support to the patient but it requires good arms, wrists and hands.

Canes and Crutches: A walking cane serves two important functions viz.

(i) It provides a means to transfer the weight of the weak limb and

(ii) It helps in maintaining the good balance while walking.

The crutches provides the best support to the patient's wrists and elbows than canes or walkers. The crutches are of two types:

(i) Forearm crutches, and

(ii) Axillary crutches.

Forearm Crutch: It is designed specifically to provide the best support to forearm above the wrist. It has a vertical extension which extends above the wrist and secured well by means of cuff or collar.

Whenever one crutch is used, it should be used on the side opposite to weak leg and when two crutches are used patient should be instructed to move forward with his left leg and right crutch followed by right leg and left crutch respectively.

Axillary Crutches: These are either made of wooden or aluminum. These provide maximum support to both wrists and elbows. The adjustable crutches are preferred since they offer better and perfect fitting.

The patient lifters are used to lift the patient.

Urology and Incontinence Supplies

The containers should be employed to collect the urine. These are called as urinals. The urinals differ in shape according to male or female use. They are made of plastics or white enamel ware.

The male condom catheters and female external catheters are designed to be worn by the patient. Catheters are used to collect the urine from the patient who are unable to void naturally e.g. Foley catheter.

An urinary bags are of two types viz.: (i) Leg bags and (ii) Night urinary collection bags.

An ambulatory patient uses the leg bag which is available in different size and capacity. The capacity of night urine collection bag is 7 litres. These bags hangs from the side of the bed or the back of the wheelchair.

Various forms of the incontinence pants for men and women are available. These pants are made of soft, flexible fabric with inner rubber or plastic coating.

The rectal tubes are used for the removal of faeces or gases from the rectum.

Ostomy Appliances: An ostomy is a surgical operation by which some part of intestine or urinary tract is removed from the patient and the open ends of the tube are brought to abdominal wall. A stoma or artificial opening is made surgically, through which the faeces or urine passes.

The karaya gum powder and other barrier pastes are used to fill the irregularities in the skin surface to prevent leakage. The deodorant drops or sprays are applied on the outside of the appliance.

Phototherapy: Phototherapy light is essential for the treatment of neonatal jaundice.

Respiratory Therapy: The steam vaporizer provides the hot steam therapy for the relief of upper respiratory illnesses such as colds, sinusitis etc.

Aerosols and nebulisers are used for administration of antibiotics directly to the site of infection. Ventilators, portable oxygen tanks and oxygen concentrator are useful for providing oxygen therapy.

QUESTIONS

1. What are diagnostic instruments ? Name various diagnostic instruments.
2. What is C.T. scan ?
3. What do you know about biopsy ?
4. Write a note on equipments for drains and splints.
5. Write in short about "Laser" and "Lithotripsy."
6. Prepare a list of surgical instruments and give the use of each.
7. Name various health accessories used in the hospital.

***

9

PHARMACY AND THERAPEUTIC COMMITTEE

The perfect choice of drugs from numerous available drugs for use in the hospital is an important administrative and therapeutic tool. Between 1920-1940, there was not much establishment in drug therapy, however definite standards for improving drug therapy were established during this period. The American Medical Association had established the rules to guide the manufacturers as well as physicians.

After this period there were new inventions of large number of antibiotics of varying activity, potency and toxicity. Because of these variations, it was necessary for the hospital to develop the method to bring the best drug for the treatment of hospitalised patients. This was achieved by the formation of a good Pharmacy and Therapeutic Committee.

The Pharmacy and Therapeutic Committee

It is an advisory group of medical staff and serves as the organizational line of communication between the medical staff and pharmacy department. The committee consists of physicians, pharmacists and other health professionals. It is a body of the medical staff and administration of hospital to recommend the matters related to therapeutic use of drugs.

Purpose of the Committee

The committee has two main purposes:

1. **Advisory:** The committee recommends to adopt the policies or help in the preparation of policies regarding evaluation, selection and therapeutic use of drugs.
2. **Educational:** The committee recommends or helps in the preparation of programmes through which the need of the professional staff for complete current knowledge cn matters related to drugs and their use will be fulfilled.

Organisation of the Committee

To carry out the functions of P and T committee efficiently, a proper organizational structure is necessary. However the composition and operation of P and T committee varies from hospital to hospital depending on its size and location.

I. The P and T committee should be composed of
   (a) At least three physicians,
   (b) A pharmacist,
   (c) A nurse representative.

II. A chairman should be appointed from amongst the physician representatives. A pharmacist usually works as a secretary.

III. The meeting of the committee should be at least six times per year and whenever necessary.

IV. An agenda should be prepared by the secretary and submitted to the committee members within sufficient time before the meeting.

V. The secretary should prepare the minutes of the committee meeting and maintain the permanent records for the hospital.

VI. The recommendations of the committee should be presented to the medical staff for its adoption or recommendation.

Functions and Scope of the Committee

1. To advise the medical staff and hospital administration in matters relating to the use of drugs.
2. To establish and develop suitable educational schemes to improve the hospital's professional staff on the matters related to the use of drugs.
3. To develop and compile formulary of drugs and prescriptions accepted for use in hospital. It also minimises the duplication of the same type of drugs or products.
4. To study problems related to the distribution and administration of drugs used in hospital.
5. To review adverse drug interactions occurring in hospital.
6. To initiate and promote the studies on drug use and review the results of such studies.
7. To recommend drugs which need to be stocked in the hospital patient care areas.
8. To advise the pharmacy in the implementatio.ı of effective drug distribution and control procedures.

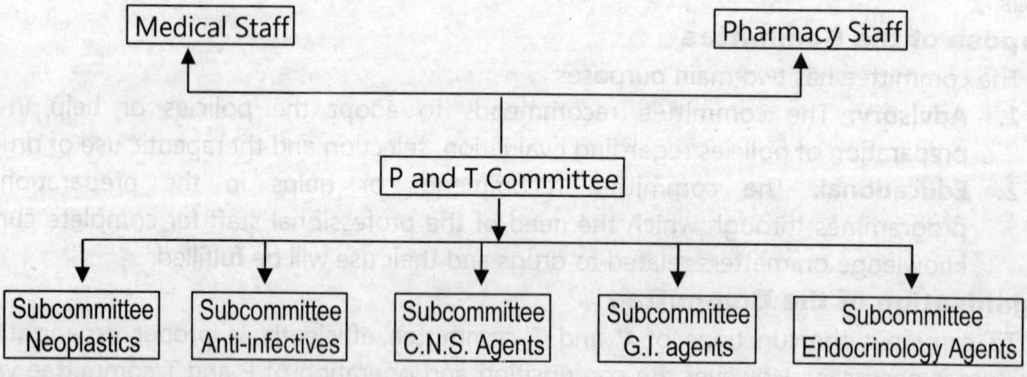

Committee Agenda

A typical agenda consists of the following:

1. Minutes of the previous meeting.
2. Review of the specified section of the formulary for updating and deletion of products.
3. Listing of new drugs which have become commercially available.
4. Investigational drugs currently in use in the hospital.
5. Review of adverse drug reactions reported in the hospital since the last meeting.
6. Drug safety in the hospital.

Policies of the Committee

The use of drugs in hospital is controlled by establishing different policies. Following are the examples of thoroughness required:

[A] Proposal of a new drug for the Hospital Formulary should be submitted on a Formulary Request Form to the Pharmacy Department.

[B] Drugs evaluated and approved by the committee are be assigned to one of the following categories.

1. Formulary drug: An FDA approved drug which is essential for good patient care and with well established usage.
2. Drugs approved on a conditional Trial Period.

A drug approved by FDA for general use but which the committee will evaluate for a 6 or 12 months period before final consideration.

3. Specialised formulary Drug: FDA approved drug recommonded for use in specialised patient care.
4. Investigational Drugs: FDA approved drug for a specific use by its principal investigator and designated associates. Such drugs are not commercially available.

[C] Drugs which do not qualify under the four categories listed above are considered as "Non-Formulary Drugs" and will not be stocked in the pharmacy.

[D] The committee is responsible for the rules and regulations which activities govern pharmaceutical company representatives in hospital.

[E] The pharmacy department is authorised to dispense drugs according to policies and procedures of the committee.

[F] The pre-signing of blank prescriptions or drug orders is prohibited.

[G] Drug Recall: After receiving the drug recall notice, all the drugs will be removed and replaced. This information is sent to all the staff and respective hospital departments.

The Role of Pharmacy and Therapeutic Committee in Drug Safety

The responsibility of hospital pharmacist increases proportionately with the vast increase of therapeutic agents. Along with increased responsibility, the capability of insuring safety in the handling and administration of drugs must increase.

Hence the function of drug safety in the hospital will be the responsibility of the committee. The following are the guidelines for the committee in achieving Drug Safety in the hospital.

1. Hospital should employ a qualified registered pharmacist (atleast B. pharm.) as a chief pharmacist and others who are Diploma holders.
2. Hospital should not permit personnel without a pharmacy degree to dispense drugs.
3. Sufficient number of qualified personnel must be employed in the hospital.
4. Hospital should provide adequate and safe work space and storage facilities for the pharmacy.
5. Adequate number of equipments in good condition should be provided for safe practice of pharmacy.
6. Automatic stop order regulation should be there in the hospital.
7. A drug formulary should be there in hospital which is periodically revised and kept upto date.
8. The poisonous materials should be kept separately from non-poisonous materials in the pharmacy and nursing stations.

9. The external use preparations should be separated from internal use preparations in the pharmacy and in the wards.
10. The hospital should allow the chief pharmacist to engage in teaching programme to familiarise the nursing and residential staff with new drugs.
11. No one should be permitted other than registered pharmacist into the pharmacy "after hours."
12. All nursing drug stations should be periodically inspected for removing the deteriorated and outdated drugs.
13. Adequate reference library should be provided for the pharmacy and nursing staff.

The Committee's Role in Adverse Drug Reaction Program

It is the committee's responsibility for developing and instituting a procedure for the reporting of adverse drug reaction.

An adverse drug reaction can be defined as any pathological condition caused by overdosage; hypersensitivity; allergy; or injury, from improper technique of administration, use of the wrong drug, error in compounding, labelling or packaging, or from other errors in the manufacture of drug for use in the hospital.

The committee should prepare an adverse drug reaction report form. Every case of adverse drug reaction must be reported by attending physician.

1. Name of Patient

ADVERSE DRUG REACTION REPORT

1. Name of the Drug ......
2. Type of Reaction ......
3. Age ...... 4. Sex .... 5. Weight ......
6. Daily dose ...... 7. Date (a) started ...... (b) Ended ......
8. Source of drug ...... (a) Prescription ...... (c) Other ......
(b) Over the counter ......

The Role of Committee in Developing Emergency Drug Lists

In most emergencies, time is of great importance, hence emergency drug boxes containing drugs and supplies should be readily available at the bedside at all times. The P and T Committee should develop a list of supplies and drugs which should be in an emergency box and instruct the pharmacist and nursing supervisor to have the box ready for use at all the times.

After the contents of the box has been established and the responsibility for its stocking assigned, the units should be prepared and placed in each ward, in the clinic and in the special procedures room.

QUESTIONS

1. What is P and T committee ? Give its purpose.
2. Write in brief about the organization of a pharmacy and therapeutic committee.
3. What are the policies of P and T committee ?
4. Describe the role of P and T committee in drug safety and adverse drug reactions.
5. Give the functions of PTC.

***

10

HOSPITAL FORMULARY SYSTEM

Hospital formulary is defined as a list of drugs used in the hospital. The hospital formulary should be revised continuously and it reflects the current clinical judgement of the medical staff.

The hospital formulary system is a method or an ongoing process by which hospital's medical staff in consultation with P and T committee evaluates and selects drugs from that it considers most useful in patient care among the numerous drugs available in the market.

Reasons for the Disfavour of Hospital Formulary System

1. The hospital formulary system deprives the physician to prescribe and obtain the brand of his choice.
2. This system does not reduce the cost of drugs to the patient because most institutions purchase large volumes of drugs at reduced rates (concessional, discount, or any scheme) but do not pass on to the patient any reduction in their cost.
3. The system allows for the purchase of inferior quality drugs, especially in institutions where there is no staff pharmacist.
4. The system at many times permits the pharmacist to act as the sole judge of which brand of drug is to be purchased and dispensed.

In an institution with an active and well formed P and T committee, the above reasons will disappear. The committee will select the drugs at most economic cost both to the hospital as well as to the patient.

Organisation of the Formulary

There are four primary objectives of the formulary:

1. To provide the hospital staff, the information on which drugs have been selected for use in the hospital by the committee.
2. Formulary provides the staff basic therapeutic information about each selected drug.
3. It also provides information on hospital policies and procedures governing the use of drugs.
4. It gives special information about drugs such as drug dosing rules, sodium content of various drugs, and hospital approved abbreviations.

In respect of above objectives, the formulary should consist of three main parts.

I. Information on hospital policies and procedures concerning drugs.

II. Drug products listing and

III. Special information.

Formulary Appearance

The appearance of the formulary must be as follows

1. Title page.
2. Names and titles of the members of P and T committee.
3. Table of contents.
4. Information regarding the policies and procedures concerning the drugs in the hospital.
5. Products accepted for use in the hospital.

   It must contain the list of items added and deleted from the previous edition, generic-brand name, and table of therapeutic index with relative cost codes.
6. **Appendix:** It includes the rules for calculating paediatric dose, body surface area, schedules of standard drug administration times.

Legal Aspects of Formulary System

In a hospital, the physician has to write the prescription and sign it in the Doctor's order book. It is the only legal prescription and the pharmacist then dispenses it. But if the physician write the chemical name of the drug then the pharmacist may dispense the brand in his judgement which meets the therapeutic need.

But the problem will arise when the formulary system is put into effect in the hospital and the prescriber due to his habit uses the proprietary names of the drug. To avoid such complications different methods are used in hospital for obtaining prior medical consent to the operation of hospital formulary system.

1. To use printed wordings on the prescription form

e.g. (a) Generic names only

(b) Dispense in accordance with the hospital formulary.

In some hospitals the consent statement is often followed by 'Yes' or 'No' statement so that the physician gets the option of prescribing specific drugs.

2. To incorporate in the basic policy and procedures of the hospital or in the rules and regulations and
3. To express the policies and procedures governing the hospital formulary system in a separate set of papers and request all physicians to accept the procedure and sign the document.

Reasons for the Need of Hospital Formulary

The need of hospital formulary system is increasing now-a-days because of:

1. the increase in number of new drugs in market.
2. the increased influence of advertising and unscientific "scientific" drug literature.

3. competition in marketing practices of Pharmaceutical Industry.
4. the increased complications of untoward effects of the new drugs.
5. the feeling of public that health professions provide best possible care at the lowest possible cost.

Guiding Principles of Hospital Formulary System

The following principles will serve as a guide to all those utilizing the formulary system:

1. The medical staff of the hospital should appoint a P and T committee and outline its scope, purpose, organization and function.
2. The formulary system should be sponsored by medical staff based upon recommendations of P and T committee.
3. The medical staff should adopt the written policies and procedures of the formulary system.
4. Drugs should be included in the formulary by their non-proprietary names and should be prescribed by the same name.
5. Limiting the number of drugs available from pharmacy can produce substantial patient care and financial benefits. These benefits can be greatly increased by using generic equivalents.

Generic equivalent: The drugs containing identical active components e.g. two brands of tetracycline.

Therapeutic equivalent: The drugs differing in composition but having very similar pharmacologic or therapeutic effect e.g. two different antacid products.

6. The management of the hospital should inform all the medical and nursing staff about the existence of the formulary system, procedures of operation of the system and any changes in those procedures. Copies of the formulary must be readily available at all times.
7. Provision should be made for the use of drugs not included in the formulary, by the medical staff.
8. The pharmacist should be responsible for specifications as to the quality, quantity and source of supply of all drugs used in the diagnosis and treatment of patients.

Guiding Principles for Admission or Deletion of Drugs in the Formulary

Following criteria should be taken into consideration for admission or deletion of drugs in formulary:

1. Whether the medical staff consider the drug to be of proved clinical value based on their experience with it.
2. Drug must be recognised by the pharmacopoeias and formularies approved under Drugs and Cosmetic Act and Rules thereunder.
3. The manufacturer of the drug should have the licence under Drugs and Cosmetic Rules and should not have been punished for any serious offence under any law of Drugs and Medicines.

4. No drug or preparation of secret composition should be admitted in the formulary.
5. No drug or preparation containing many ingredients should be admitted if the similar therapeutic effect can be obtained by the use of single ingredient preparation.

Preparation of the Formulary

The first step in the development of a formulary for any hospital is to form a competent Pharmacy and Therapeutic committee. The committee then decides on the following:

1. What type of publication will be most suitable for the hospital ?
   (a) A hospital's own formulary or
   (b) A simple list of drugs or
   (c) A purchased formulary service.
2. Fixation of rules which the committee may use to evaluate drugs for admission to the formulary.
3. If the formulary is to be prepared, decision must be taken on its contents in each section such as:
   (a) Prescription writing.
   (b) Use of drugs.
   (c) Table of metric weights and apothecary and household equivalents.
   (d) Tables of common laboratory values.
   (e) Section on calculation of doses for children.
   (f) Pharmacological index.
   (g) Section on reagents.
4. The type of format of the formulary
   (a) Size.
   (b) Loose leaf or bounded.
   (c) Printed or mimeographed.
   (d) Extent of categorization and indexing.

Formulary and Drug List

Usually people use these two terms synonymous to each other. But in fact these are not. A formulary consists of a list of therapeutic agents by their generic names followed by the data on various aspects such as strength, form, posology, toxicology, use and quantity to be dispensed. Whereas a drug list consists of a list of therapeutic agents by their generic names followed by data on strength and form only. Hence the formulary is more informative publication than a drug fist.

If a formulary is to be prepared, whether a private formulary for hospital or to subscribe the perpetual drug monograph service such as National formulary of India. Both the types have their own advantages.

Private Formulary	National Formulary
1. It is prepared by the hospitals own clinical staff.	1. It is prepared by nation's outstanding clinicians, pharmacologists and pharmacists.
2. The information given under each monograph is subject to local needs. It may include related clinical matters.	2. Each monograph contains physical and chemical properties, pharmacologic responses, uses, toxicology, posology, preparations and contraindications.
3. It is published in a more convenient size and format.	3. Since too many drugs are listed the size of formulary is big.
4. Drugs may be added or deleted with greater frequency.	4. Drugs are added or deleted with less frequency.

Content of Formulary

The content of formulary depends completely on those who are responsible for its publication. But it is most important to include a section of prescription writing in the formulary which is useful for young physicians joining as trainee staff. The following are the guidelines for prescription writing.

All prescriptions must be written clearly in a medical order which indicates the following information:

Name and address of the patient,
The date,
The Medicines prescribed,
(It should be written in the terminology given in the formulary)
The strength of the medicines prescribed (in the metric system),
The total amount to be dispensed should be clearly indicated.

The signs, containing the instructions to the patient should be in clear and simple terminology. If refill of the preparation is needed, then for how many times, should be indicated and if not, preparation will not be refilled by the pharmacist. The prescription for narcotic drugs must indicate the narcotic number of the prescribing physician and patient's name in addition to above information. All the prescriptions should be signed by the concerned physician. Other informative data regarding the laboratory values, tables for calculation of percentages and dosages, tables of heights and weights and formulae and such other data, that P and T committee considers useful must also be included in the formulary.

The Format, Size and Appearance of Formulary

The format of the formulary is most important because on it depends the daily use and publishing cost of the formulary.

Facilities

The hospital pharmacist collects the formularies of various hospitals and then decides the format of the formulary. After publication of the formulary, two copies need to be sent to the American Society of Hospital Pharmacist.

Depending on the local need of the hospital, the formulary should be published in specific size so that it will be convenient for use to the physicians. The formulary of smaller size will always be preferred.

The appearance of the formulary means whether the formulary should be in form of loose - leaf or bound and printed or mimeographed. A loose - leaf formulary can be kept upto-date easily than a bound type formulary. A bound type formulary requires more frequently revisions. A loose-leaf formulary can be revised easily by inserting and distributing the printed pages. In case of bound formulary many ranges are there from paper to cardboard or plastic, or leather. The National Formulary of India is a card-board bound volume.

QUESTIONS

1. Define Hospital formulary. Give reasons for the disfavour of hospital formulary system.
2. What are the objectives of the formulary?
3. Why is hospital formulary, system needed in the hospital? Give its guiding principles.
4. Write notes on:
   (i) Preparation of formulary.
   (ii) Contents of formulary.
   (iii) Addition or deletion of drugs in the formulary.
   (iv) Format and size of the formulary.

***

11

DRUG INFORMATION SPECIALIST AND SERVICES

This chapter aims to describe the concept of Drug Information Services so that the pharmacist or student can understand its purpose, scope and functions.

In health care delivery, drugs are used as tools by the physicians. In the drug use process, these are handled by other health care professionals, such as pharmacist, nursing staff etc. and the patients consume the drugs for their medical care. For proper use of medications by physicians, pharmacist, nurses and patients require information about drugs. With rapid advancement in medical and biological sciences, a huge information about drugs, diseases, diagnostic procedures, pathological findings etc. has emerged out. Availability of large number of drug formulations, introduction of new drugs and dosage forms, complexity of multiple drug use, all these factors point out the need of information about drugs for their rational selection and utilization.

Over the last 25 years, the introduction of numerous new drugs has caused a massive increase in the volume of pharmaceutical and related medical literature. This proliferation has led directly to the establishment of the first drug information centre under the auspices of a pharmacist at the University of Kentucky in 1962. Later the drug information centres were established in the U.K. in Leeds and London in 1970. Some specialist services were established which lead to formation of regional-based drug information centres. In 1976 the foundation was laid for a national drug information network.

For health professionals most information about drugs is provided by industry through their Medical Service Representative (MSR), advertising, literature inserts and physician desk references. Most of the times, these sources can't provide the objective information needed by prescribes. Nursing staff and patient may not receive this information and even if they receive it is inadequate and insufficient to answer their questions. Thus there is a necessity of DIS to cater to the need of physicians, pharmacist, nurses and patients.

Pharmacist being expert on drugs is most suitable and competant professional to provide these services. Logically drug information should be a part of pharmacy practice and pharmacist/DIS/scientist. Thus one of the services provided by clinical pharmacist is DISs. Drug information is provided to variety of professionals and patients and information that needs to be provided is of varied nature. Hence there is need to establish a Drug Information Centre.

Need for Drug Information Centre (DIC)

1. Bank of Therapeutic Information: Many physicians require information for taking proper decision about drug treatment. Depending on complexity of clinical situations, the information needs to be supplied as quickly as possible by DIC in hospitals. One of the main functions of the drug information centre is to provide a bank of information on drugs both for the clinician and the clinical pharmacist.

2. Backup for Clinical Pharmacist or Assist in the Service of Clinical Pharmacist: Clinical pharmacists receive questions from other professionals pertaining to drug and this information can be obtained from DIC.

The common method for physicians to obtain information about drugs through a visit of medical representative of a pharmaceutical company. Other ways are by attending lectures, by reading advertisements in the medical literature, studying articles in medical press, product data sheets circulated by the manufacturers, reports from the committee on safety of medicines and publications, like Drug and Therapeutics Bulletin, Adverse Reactions Bulletin etc.

After choosing an appropriate therapy, advice may be needed about dose and regimens, routes of administration, possible side effects, potential interactions, how and when one should discontinue therapy.

The pharmacodynamic aspects of products are often widely publicized in data sheets by manufacturers but the pharmacokinetic aspects of the products are not so readily found. For this reason all types of drug information can be obtained from drug information centres. The clinical pharmacist can fulfil his need with the back-up of information resources but on a wider basis, the need may be met by publishing Drug-information bulletins of abstracts and reviews.

The other useful functions of drug information services are as follows:

(a) Monitoring: The adverse drug reactions and reporting to the committee on safety of medicines.

(b) Educational: Teaching should be an integral part of drug information service for undergraduate level and as part of the continuing education of pharmacists.

(c) These services enable the clinical pharmacist to function in the patient care area and to participate in decision-making about medication, patient counselling and in taking medication histories.

(d) The participation of Pharmacy and Therapeutic committee have a great influence on committee's discussions and in implementing their decisions.

(e) It also has an influence on the choice and conduct of drug therapy since such a committee rationalizes hospital medication by selecting certain products within a group e.g. Anti-depressants, antihypertensives etc. and ensuring their proper use.

(f) These services are also useful for preparing and maintaining the hospital formulary. Pharmacists engaged in DICs, prepare drug education monographs for drugs to be considered for formulary addition or deletion. DIC provides complete review of drug and can provide more objective information which is useful in formulary updating and maintenance.

Sources of Information

A drug information centre must have a good collection of source material in order to deal with questions as they arise. This should be continually updated and maintained.

The information originates from research and development. This knowledge is publicized for the first time by way of what are called as 'primary sources'. Conferences including discussion sessions are the valuable sources of primary information. From these come preprints of papers and published proceedings.

Secondary Sources of Information

It means information previously appearing in primary sources. These are usually abstracting or indexing services.

International Pharmaceutical Abstracts (IPA) covers pharmacy journals. It also covers clinical journals.

The formularies, pharmacopoeias, textbooks and journals fall in this category. Some textbooks are narrow in their coverage such as a monograph on a particular drug while others are wide ranging.

The following formularies, pharmacopoeias and text books must be available in the drug information centre.

Formularies

1. National Formulary of India (NFI).
2. British National Formulary (BNF).
3. National Formulary of America (NFA).
4. Australian Pharmaceutical Formulary (APF).

Pharmacopoeias

1. Indian Pharmacopoeia (I.P.).
2. British Pharmacopoeia (B.P.).
3. British Pharmaceutical Codex (B.P.C.).
4. European Pharmacopoeia (E.P.).
5. French Pharmaceutical Codex (F.P.C.).
6. German Pharmacopoeia (G.P.).
7. Swiss Pharmacopoeia (S.P.)
8. United States Pharmacopoeia (U.S.P.)

Journals, Periodicals and Text-Books

1. American Journal of Hospital Pharmacy
2. British Medical Journal
3. Drugs

4. Drug Intelligence and Clinical pharmacy
5. Indian journal of Medical Research
6. Indian Journal of Pharmacy
7. Indian Journal of Hospital Pharmacy
8. Journal of American Medical Association
9. Journal of Indian Medical Association
10. Journal of Clinical and Hospital Pharmacy
11. Journal of Pharmacy and Pharmacology
12. Journal of Clinical Phamacology
13. Journal of Pharmaceutical Sciences
14. Lancet
15. New England Journal of Medicine
16. Pharma Times
17. Practitioner
18. Drug Interactions
19. Eastern Pharmacist
20. Materia Medics
21. Martidale's Extra Pharmacopoeia
22. Merck Index
23. Merck Manual
24. Remington's Practice of Pharmaceutical Sciences
25. Text Book of Hospital Pharmacy
26. Theory and Practice of Industrial Pharmacy – Leon Lachman
27. Law of Drugs and Medicines – Beotra
28. Clinical Toxicology – Lee
29. Pharmcological Basis of Therapeutics – Goodman and Gilman.

Tertiary Sources of Information

The information contained in the publications under this heading usually does not answer the problems in hand but acts as a pointer to where it may be found. The dictionaries and encyclopaedias provide derivations and definitions of terms used in the literature.

A good medical dictionary and a good English language dictionary are essential to drug information centres.

The followings fall under this source of information:

1. The Chemist and Druggist Directory.
2. Indian Pharmaceutical Guide - which gives the manufacturers or suppliers catalogues and price lists.
3. Medical Register, Annual Register and Directory of Pharmaceutical Chemists.
4. Statistical tables and mathematical tables to provide scientific data.

Location of Drug Information Centre

The drug information centre or the "Pharmacy Library" should be located within the pharmacy department of the hospital. The individual using this facility is usually the pharmacist and physician. Hence at the time of spot consultation or whenever the need of mathematical or statistical tables for calculating the doses for children or old people, the physician does not need to visit the the hospital library which may be at a distant place. This saves the working time of both physician and pharmacist and helps in providing efficient service. In U.S.A. some DICs are poison control centres.

Physical Facilities

The dimensions of the pharmacy library depends on the size of the staff utilizing this library and the type of hospital and number of publications to be kept in it. The Handbook of Medical Library Practice provides the following dimensions as being useful for determining the space requirements.

1. The reading area should be 25-30 square feet per reader.
2. Each table should provide the floor space of 100 square feet for four readers and if:
   (a) Circular tables – 48 inches diameter
   (b) Rectangular tables – 36 × 60 feet
3. **Gaps:**
   (a) Between tables – Not less than 5 feet
   (b) Between tables and walls – 3 to 4 feet
4. **Shelf Space:**
   (a) Bound volumes – 4 to 5 volumes per foot of shelf
   (b) Reference tools – 3 to 4 volumes per foot of shelf

Additional space of 7 inches per 3 feet should be kept for additions and removal.

Personnel and Staffing

Pharmacist on staff of pharmacy department is drug information specialist; interested staff pharmacist, volunteers, librarian, graduate and undergraduate students.

Pharmacist is secretary and is drug information specialist in formal DIS. Formal DISs rotate staff pharmacist system – everyone has opportunity to gain DIS experience. Interested staff pharmacist can assume the role of Drug Information Specialist in absence of formal DIS. Volunteers with basic clerical abilities can be helpful in maintaining the library aspects of DIC-collection cataloging and storage of information. Liaison with the clinical pharmacist and the DIS should be established by the presence of clinical librarian - who can also take patient care and handle library. Graduate and undergraduate students are also manpower for DIS.

Each department must decide the best approach to provide information, considering departmental goals, budget and space.

Availability of Services: 24 hours.

Records and Reports: DIS should document its activity on a daily basis and periodically through out the year. Summary of monthly report would facilitate writing of annual report.

Funding of DIS: It is most important aspect of DIS program. Permanent budget or hard money sources and totally and partly funding – Department of pharmacy, medical department, library, pharmacology, schools of pharmacy, charging for DIS, fees generated through bulletin, research projects by staff, courses taught by DIS staff to other department, extended consultation are all sources for funds.

Drug Information Network: (DIN)

The ultimate goal of DIS is to promote rational drug use by professionals and the lay public and this goal can be met by DIN composed of regional DISs; that serve a given area of country. Regional centres develop satellite centres based in pharmacy department providing services in hospitals.

More practitioners and patients should receive the benefit of timely drug information which should improve medication use

Abilities: For this four levels of personnel are identified.

1. DIS director
2. DIS staff
3. Graduates and residents
4. Undergraduates.

Service Function

DIS functions as a resource of information on all aspects of drugs for health care professionals, include.

1. Collection and Storage of Information

(a) Books and monographs.

(b) Current biochemical literature (files).

(c) Mannuals and journals, medical journal advertising.

(d) Electronic data processing, Tapes, floppies etc.

These sources would not replace the pharmacist as the drug information specialist, but rather would function as tools in this service.

2. Retrieval of Stored Information

Commercially available systems produce journals covering pharmacy practice, the pharmaceutical sciences and the clinical and economical aspects of drug.

All these commercially available systems for retrieval have a significant lag time the time between original publication of article and inclusion of the article in the retrieval systems.

3. Evaluation of Information

Most distinguishing characteristic of a DIS is the evaluation of information prior to answering an inquiry or providing a consultation.

Increasing quantity and variable quality of the drug literature requires an evaluation step. This is useful in formulary system in writing of monographs.

4. Dissemination of Information

The drug information can be communicated over the telephone, in person and in writing. Both verbal and written communication skills are essential in disseminating drug information.

The specialist should answer the questions, whenever possible, rather than to provide information which pertains to it. Clinical training and experience is essential for producing clinically relevant drug information.

To increase the visibility of the service and establish contact for further consultation, the specialist should meet the head of the institution.

He must know proper questions to ask while attempting to provide information to formulate a meaningful response. He should be able to answer the questions on identification, availability and pharmaceutical compatibility. Sources for Dissemination of Informations: (1) Telephone (2) In person (3) Writing (4) Drug monograph prepared for PTC review (5) News letters, and bulletins.

Educational Activities: It is an important part of overall daily programme. DIS staff undergo daily education.

It is important to set realistic goals for students rotating through the DIS, and to make efficient use of their time. Some of the educational activities are:

1. To provide continuing education lectures and seminars to staff and health professionals.
2. To present and review interesting drug information requests at scheduled seminars.
3. To instruct undergraduate students on the effective use of resources in the DIS and
4. To prepare specific written guidelines on any aspect of drug usage for use by pharmacist, nurses and physicians in patient care areas.

The Abilities Required for a Drug Information Specialist

1. Demonstration of professional and technical competence in the evaluation, critical selection and utilization of drug literature. Presentation of the maximum relevant information with a minimal volume of pertinent supporting documentation to permit independent, informed conclusions and decisions.
2. Knowledge of institutional and extramural library facilities, literature utilization and library services.
3. Possession of verbal and written communication skills.
4. Capacity to contribute to the continuing education of all health professions.
5. Participation directly and indirectly in patient care by monitoring drug regimen.
6. Familarity with electronic data processing for information retrieval.
7. Provision of professional services to the Pharmacy and Therapeutic committee.
8. Rendering of professional judgement to bring effective pharmaceutical services into the mainstream of patient care, thus contributing to clinical pharmacy practice and the education of its practitioners.
9. Contribution to drug literature through appropriate research.

Pharmacist's ancient functions of compounding and dispensing medicine have atrofied and been displaced by the progress of the drug industry.

Organization, attitudes, communication and therapeutics are the present deficiencies of the pharmacist in the clinical environment. Pharmacist has become a guide, leader, advisor and counselor to all the people around him and are no longer just compounders and dispensors of medicine.

Drug Information Bulletin

The drug information centre could publish a booklet to communicate the recent information about the drugs to all the health professionals in the hospital; which is called as drug information bulletin (DIB).

Importance of DIB

It acts as a link between the drug information centre and health professionals. The information is communicated to physicians, pharmacists, nurses and other health professionals in the shortest possible time for application in the clinical pharmacy practice. The bulletin gives information about recent advances in medical research and the detailed information about drugs to the physician and pharmacist. It also publishes the matter in "Question-Answer" session and abstracts on "New Developments." This service helps in keeping the medical staff of the hospital alert about recent drug research and using the same in clinical practice.

QUESTIONS

1. Describe the scope and functions of the drug information services.
2. Explain the different sources of drug information.
3. Write in brief about tertiary sources of information.
4. What are the abilities required of "Drug information Specialist"?
5. What is "Drug Information Bulletin"? Give its importance.

***

12

SURGICAL DRESSINGS

The surgical dressings are used to cover the wounds to enable quick healing of wounds. These are also used for medication purpose and to absorb and retain a wide range of fluids from the blood and serous exudate of damaged tissue.

Ideal properties of the surgical dressing are as follows:

1. It should be non-adherent to skin surface.
2. It should have the maximum absorbing capacity.
3. It should be cheap and non-inflammable.
4. It should be porous to water vapour, otherwise the sweat from the surrounding skin will accumulate and delay the healing.
5. It should be free from foreign substances that cause tissue reactions such as allergy or hypersensitivity.
6. It should be capable of being sterilised by conventional methods.
7. It should be unaffected by industrial solvent such as detergents and oils.
8. It should have sufficient tensile strength.
9. It should be smooth on both the surfaces.
10. It should have constant physical properties under normal conditions of storage and use.

[I] COTTON

Category: Surgical aid. (For cleaning and swabbing wounds, preoperative skin preparation, application of medicament, supplementary absorbent pad to absorb excess wound exudate).

Description: It is white, soft, fine filament like hair appearing under the microscope as hollow, flattened and twisted bands, sıriated and slightly thickened at the edges. It is practically odourless and tasteless.

Solubility: Insoluble in ordinary solvents; soluble in ammoniated cupric oxide TS.

Purified cotton is the hairy part of the seed of cultivated varieties of Gossypium Hirsutum Linne or of other species of Gossypium (Family: Malvaceae) freed from adhering impurities, deprived of fatty matter, bleached and sterilized in its final container.

Packaging and Storage: Packages are in rolls of not more than 500 g of a continuous lap, with light weight paper running under the entire lap enclosed and sealed in a well closed container.

Labelling: Label bears a statement that the sterility cannot be guaranteed if the package bears evidence of damage or if the package has been opened previously.

Alkalinity or Acidity: About log of cotton is thoroughly saturated with 100 ml of recently boiled and cooled water. Then with the aid of glass rod press out two 25 ml portions of water into white porcelain dishes. To one portion add 3 drops of phenolphthalein and to the other portion add 1 drop of methyl orange. No pink colour develops in either portion.

Residue on Ignition: Place about 5 g accurately weighed, in a porcelain or platinum dish and moisten with diluted sulphuric acid. Gently heat the cotton until it is charred, then ignite more strongly until the carbon is completely consumed. Cool in a desiccator, weigh and calculate the percentage of residue. Not more than 0.2% residue remains.

Water soluble substances: Not more than 0.35%

Fatty matter: Not more than 0.7%

Fibre Length and Absorbency: Remove cotton from its wrappings and condition it for not less than 4 hours in a standard atmosphere of 65% relative humidity at 21°C before determining the fibre length and absorbency.

Fibre Length: Not less than 60% of fibres, by weight, are 12.5 mm or greater in length and not more than 10% of the fibres by weight are 6.25 mm or less in length.

Absorbency: The cotton retains not less than 24 times its weight of water.

Sterility: It should satisfy the sterility test.

[II] GAUZE

Absorbent Gauze (Absorbent Cotton Gauze).

Category: Surgical aid (for pre-operative preparation, for cleansing and swabbing), for direct-wound dressing.

It is a white cotton cloth of various thread counts and weights, lengths and widths supplied in the form of rolls or folds. It is in the form of plain woven cloth.

Packaging and storage: In a well closed container such that the sterility of contents is maintained until the package is opened for use. Waxed paper should not be used for any wrapping in contact with gauze as it reduces the absorbency.

Labelling: Label should indicate (1) Its type or thread count, length and width and the number of pieces contained. (2) "Non-sterilized"or "Not sterilized" and if "sterile" then contents may not be sterile if the package bears evidence of damage or has been previously opened. (3) The name of manufacturer, packer or distributor.

Identification test: It produces violet colour after treatment with iodinated zinc chloride solution.

Threads Per Stated Length: Warp; average 73/10 cm. weft; average 57 per 10 cm.

Weight per unit area: Average 15 g per m^2.

Absorbency: The sinking time is not more than 10 seconds.

Acidity or alkalinity: The extract with water does not show pink colour with phenolphthalein but shows yellow colour with methyl orange.

Water soluble substances: Not more than 0.5%.

Ether soluble substances: Not more than 0.5%.

Sulphated ash: Not more than 0.75%.

Sterilization: It may be sterilized by autoclaving, hot air oven or by ionizing radiations.

Absorbent Ribbon Gauze: (Unmedicated ribbon gauze)

It consists of cloth of plain weave supplied in ribbons of various widths and length. The threads are of cotton or rayon.

Its absorbency reduces by medication, prolonged storage or exposure to heat.

Uses: It is used to pack sinus, throat, dental cavities and open infected wounds to assist healing. It swells in use, which should be considered while packing small cavities.

Gauze and Cotton Tissue: (Absorbent Gauze Tissue)

It consists of thick layer of absorbent cotton wool enclosed in gauze in tubular form.

Standards: These are similar to that of Absorbent Gauze.

Uses: It is used as an absorbent and protective pad with or without an additional dressing. It is also used as burns dressing on non-adherent layer.

Gauze Swab: It consists of absorbent cotton gauze type 13, light or absorbent cotton and viscose gauze type 1 folded into square or rectangles of 8-ply with no cut edges exposed.

Filmated gauze swab consists of gauze swab with thin layer of absorbent cotton enclosed within.

Non-woven Swab: It consists of non-woven viscose fabric folded 4-ply, alternative to gauze swabs.

Use: General purpose swabbing and cleansing. It absorbs more quickly than gauze.

[III] BANDAGES

(A) Retention Bandages

The retention bandages are of two types:

(i) Non-stretch fabric, and

(ii) Stretch fabric,

Non-stretch Fabric Retention Bandages

1. Triangular Calico Bandage

It consists of triangular shaped piece of unbleached cotton cloth of plain weave.

It is clean and reasonably free from weaving defects, cotton leaf and shell.

Uses: It is used as a sling. If the bandage is likely to be in contact with area of broken skin, it should be sterilized before use.

2. Domette Bandage

It consists of fabric of plain weave in which the warp threads are of cotton and weft threads are of wool.

Uses: It is used mainly for orthopaedic purposes where a higher degree of warmth, support and protection is required. These qualities are provided by heavy wool weft.

3. Open-wove Bandage: (Cambric Bandage)

It consists of cotton cloth of plain weave.

Uses: Protection and retention of absorbent dressings, support for minor strains, sprains. It is also used to secure splints.

Type 1 bandage is known as open wove bandage.

Type 2 bandage is known as medium quality and

Type 3 bandage is known as hospital quality.

Stretch Fabric Retention Bandages

1. Cotton Conforming Bandage

It consists of cotton cloth of plain weave, treated to impart some elasticity to warp and weft.

Uses: It is used to protect dressings and hold them in place at difficult positions such as joints.

2. Polyamide and Cellulose Contour Bandage: (Nylon and viscose stretch Bandage)

Fabric, plain weave containing warp of polyamide filament and the weft of cotton or viscose. The edges are fast with continuous length. It is used for retention of dressings.

Following are the bandages used for retention of dressings on the limbs, trunk and abdomen.

(a) Elasticated Tubular Bandage

(b) Foam padded Elasticated Surgical Tubular Stockinette.

(B) Support and Compression Bandages

1. Crepe Bandage

It consists of fabric of plain weave in which the warp is of cotton and wool threads and weft is of cotton threads.

Uses: It is used in the treatment of sprains and strains and other condition which require light support. It is also used for correctional purposes and as compression over paste bandages for varicose veins.

The elasticity of the bandage is lost during its use which can be restored by washing the bandage in hot soapy water.

2. Cotton Crepe Bandage

A fabric of plain weave in which the warp threads are of crepe twisted cotton and the weft threads are of cotton and/or rayon.

Uses: Same as crepe bandage.

3. Cotton Stretch Bandage

It is a fabric of plain weave having the warp threads are of crepe twisted cotton and weft threads of cotton. It is stretch bandage which is lighter than cotton crepe bandage.

Uses: Same as crepe bandage.

4. Cotton and Rubber Elastic Bandage

It is a fabric of plain weave having the warp threads of cotton and rubber and weft threads of cotton.

Uses: Same as crepe bandage.

5. Elastic Adhesive Bandage

It is a woven fabric, elastic in warp (crepe twisted cotton threads) and weft of cotton and rayon threads spread with adhesive mass containing zinc oxide.

Uses: It is used as compression for chronic leg ulcers. It is also used as compression and support for fractured ribs, clavicles, swollen or sprained joints.

(C) Medicated Bandages

1. Zinc Paste Bandage

It is cotton fabric of plain weave impregnated with suitable paste containing zinc oxide. It requires additional bandaging.

The paste composition is:

Zinc oxide	180 g
Gelatine	160 g
Glycerol	255 g
Calcium chloride (dihydrate)	115 g
Boric acid	20 g
Water to make	1000 g

Content of zinc oxide in the paste - Not less than 6%

Packaging: It should be enclosed in sealed packages which prevent the entry of moisture.

Uses: It is used to support and prevent the swelling of fractured limbs after the removal of plaster. It is also used to support varicose veins and for the treatment of phlebitis, ulcers, varicose eczemas and oedema of the legs.

Example: Zincaband®.

2. Zinc Paste and Coal Tar Bandage

It is a cotton fabric of plain weave impregnated with a suitable paste containing coal tar and zinc oxide. It also requires additional bandaging.

Uses: It is used in treatment of skin disorders such as leg ulcers, neurodermatitis, chronic vesicular eczemas.

Examples: Tarband® coltapaste®.

3. Zinc Paste and Ichthammol Bandage

It is cotton fabric of plain weave impregnated with suitable paste containing zinc oxide and Ichthammol.

Uses: In the treatment of leg ulcers, chronic dermatitis and varicose eczemas.

Example: Ichthaband® Icthopaste®.

4. Plaster of Paris Bandage: (Plaster of Paris Dressing)

It is a cotton cloth impregnated with dried calcium sulphate (mixture of amorphous and crystalline forms) and suitable adhesives so that calcium sulphate remains adherent to the fabric.

Content of calcium sulphate - Not less than 85%.

Packaging: It should be enclosed in containers which prevent access of moisture and damage by pressure.

Uses: It is used for immobilization and splinting of fractures and for construction of body support. In orthopaedic surgery it is used for immobilization, support and correction splinting.

Only clean water should be used to wet the bandage before its application to avoid the infection of wounds under the bandage.

(IV) ADHESIVE TAPES

The surgical adhesive tapes are of three types:

(a) Permeable,

(b) Semipermeable, and

(c) Impermeable or occlusive.

(A) Permeable Surgical Adhesive Tapes

1. Zinc Oxide surgical Adhesive Tape (Zinc Oxide plaster)

It is a fabric of plain weave having warp and weft threads of cotton and/or rayon spread with an adhesive containing zinc oxide.

Uses: For securing dressings and immobilising small areas.

2. Elastic Surgical Adhesive Tape (Elastic Adhesive plaster)

It is woven fabric, elastic in warp (Crepe-twisted cotton threads), weft of cotton and/or rayon threads spread with adhesive mass containing zinc oxide.

Use: For securing dressings.

Example: Flexoplast® Elastoplast®.

(B) Semipermeable Surgical Adhesive Tapes

Semipermeable Waterproof Plastic Surgical Adhesive Tape: It is water impermeable, air and water vapour permeable plastic film spread with an adhesive mass.

Use: It is used for covering dressings and appliances where free passage of air and water vapour but exclusion of water is required. For covering possible sites of infection. It is used for preparation of water proof microporous plastic wound dressings.

(C) Impermeable or Occlusive Surgical Adhesive Tapes

Impermeable Plastic Surgical Adhesive Tape: It consists of water impermeable plastic film spread with an adhesive mass.

Use: It is used for securing dressings, covering site of infection where exclusion of air, water and water vapour is required.

Test for Sterility of Surgical Dressings and Sutures

The B.P.C. 1973 describes the test for sterility of surgical dressings and sutures as below:

The surgical dressing and suture must have been subjected to properly applied and monitored sterilization process.

Method

(A) Testing area

The test must be carried out under aseptic conditions in sterile area. The condition may be achieved by using laminar flow.

(B) Sample

(i) If sample consists of numerous homogeneous items e.g. individually wrapped dressings or sealed containers of suture, the items should be divided into three equal groups to perform the repeat test, if required, from each group of previously unopened item.

(ii) In case of dressings, if homogeneous item is too small, whole of the item is used if it is larger, then it is divided into equal portions.

(iii) In case of suture whole of the strand in the container should be used for the test.

(C) Culture media

Tryptone – Soya broth is recommended for use in test.

Composition

Tryptone	17 g
Soya peptone	3g
Anhydrous dextrose	2.5 g
Sodium chloride	5.0 g
Dipotassium hydrogen Phosphate	2.5 g
Distilled water	to 1000 ml

Dissolve the solids in water by heating on water bath. Adjust the pH of solution to 7.3 ± 0.1. Filter the, solution when it is hot through filter paper into different sized containers (as required). Close the containers and sterilize them by autoclaving at 121°C for 15 minutes.

Test procedure for other than paraffin gauze dressings

1. Quantities to be used in Test

(a) Culture media : Use the volume prescribed in the individual monograph

(b) Test items : Take three test portions each of

1 g dressing : unwoven material and

10 cm^2 dressing : woven material

Repeat same procedure, if re-test is necessary.

Inoculation of Medium: Inoculate the containers of selected medium (tryptone soya broth) with test portions.

Incubation: After inoculation, incubate the containers at 32°C ± 2°C for 10 days and observe them for growth of microorganisms at regular intervals.

Test Procedure for Non-absorbable Sutures

Same procedure mentioned above with following modifications.

1. Quantities to be used in the test

(a) Culture media : Use 50 ml portions of the medium.

(b) Test items : Use a whole strand from freshly opened container

2. Incubation: Incubate for 12 days.

Controls of the Test

(1) The adequacy of aseptic transfer techniques must be established by performing the test simultaneously with control items which are identical to test items.

(2) The effectiveness of culture medium in the presence and absence of sample items (fertility test) must be established.

Elimination of Antimicrobial Property: If the item under test shows the antimicrobial property (negative fertility test), then it should be eliminated by: (a) including a specific inactivator in the culture medium or (b) using membrane filtration technique to remove antimicrobial agent.

Interpretation of Results: The table given below indicates suitable interpretation of results of test for sterility. If there is failure to comply with requirements of test, the batch should be rejected.

Number of Packages or Containers in Batch	Number to be taken
Surgical dressings:	10% or 4 packages whichever is greater.
≯ 100 packages	
100-500	10
> 500	2% or 20 packages whichever is greater.
Sutures:	
≯ 1000	2% or 5 strands whichever is greater.
For each additional 1000 strands	An additional strands upto maximum total of 40.

Growth of Microorganisms in Containers Inoculated with Test Portions

1st Test	1st Retest	2nd Retest	Decision
No growth	–	–	Pass
	No growth	–	Pass
Growth in 1 container	Growth in more than 1 container	–	Fail
	Growth of same micro-organism in 1 container	–	Fail
	Growth of different micro-organism in 1 container	No growth	Pass
		Growth in 1st or more containers	Fail
Growth in 2 containers	No growth	–	Pass
	Growth in 1 or more containers.	–	Fail
Growth in more than 2 containers	–	–	Fail

Other Hospital Supplies

The equipments needed for the administration of parenteral drugs include syringes, canulas and final filtration mechanisms. These devices must be sterile, pyrogen free and free from particulate matter.

In 1896, Karl Schneider, a mechanic in Paris invented an all glass syringe with a cylindrical piston ground to fit a graduated glass barrel. Around 1925, the Luer Lok syringe was developed by Dickinson. This syringe has a thread inside the metal tip that engages the rim of the needle.

There are four categories of syringe tips.

1. **Luer-Lok Tip:** It is stronger and permanently attached to the syringe.
2. **Luer Slip Tip:** These do not lock in place. Due to pressure of injection, it may get displaced.
3. **Eccentric Tip:** It is used when needle is to be kept as parallel to the field of injection as possible.
4. **Catheter Tip:** It is not used for injection but commonly used for irrigation.

Types of Syringes

These are classified on the basis of their composition as:

(i) Glass reusable,

(ii) Glass disposable, and

(iii) Plastic disposable.

Disposable syringes are intended for one time use only. It is a standard practice to use disposable syringes for injection. The desirability of one syringe over the other depends on followings:

(i) Cost.

(ii) Product packaging.

(iii) Ability to read dosage measurement

(iv) Needle sharpness.

(v) Safety during and disposability after use.

Syringes are available in sizes from 1 ml to 60 ml and all have the design of round plunger or piston within a barrel. For reusable syringes the glass plunger is ground to fit a given barrel exactly. The barrel of the syringe is graduated in millilitres. In the design of syringes for small volumes (1 ml) the barrel is long and slender to achieve greater accuracy in measuring volume.

Insulin syringes are graduated in units of insulin (40, 80, 100 units per ml). Tuberculin syringes have capacities of 1 ml and a volume of 0.05 ml can be measured with accuracy.

Glass Disposable Syringes: These cost less than glass reusable ones, but more than those made from plastic. Compared to plastic syringes, glass disposable syringes have the advantage of ease in handling. When injections must be stored, disposable glass syringes are preferred.

Plastic Syringes: These are made from either polyethylene or polypropylene plastic and are available as sterile packaged items. They are sterilized after packaging with either ethylene oxide or radiations. Only polypropylene plastic syringes can be sterilised in an autoclave.

Maintenance of I.V. lines

- Inspect regularly for swelling, or signs of infection.
- Keep site clean and dry.
- Consider resiting the canula after 72 hours.

- Change administration sets within 72 hours.
- Wipe the hub of the cannula with an alcohol impregnated swab before attaching the administration set.

Central Venous Catheters

Various types of central venous catheters are used for a variety of parenteral medications such as total parenteral nutrition solutions, cancer chemotherapy, longterm antibiotic therapy and blood components. The length of time the central venous catheter remains in place varies from days to months or years. When these catheters are not in use, they require heparinization i.e. they are filled with heparin-lock flush solution to maintain the patency of catheter lumen.

Indwelling Catheters

The prolonged intravenous therapy needs multiple punctures of the veins, which can be avoided by using these plastic catheters. These catheters are made from polyvinyl chloride, teflon and polyethylene. These should be removed within 48 hours of insertion. These should be adiopaque, so that these can be observed on X-ray films. The choice of catheter depends on time and purpose of infusion. Three types of these catheters are available.

1. **Plain Plastic Catheter:** These are used in emergency situations when superficial veins are unavailable. It is used without needle and inserted into vein by surgical incision.

2. **Catheter Outside Needle:** The catheter accompanies the needle into the vein during vein puncture. After insertion in the vein, the catheter hub is held in place and the needle is removed and discarded.

   The plastic catheter remains in the vein. The administration set is then connected with it. It is commonly used for percutaneous I.V. infusions.

3. **Catheter inside Needle:** It consists of stainless steel needle with plastic tubing inside its lumen. After vein puncture the plastic catheter is advanced into the vein.

Urinary Catheters

Type of Catheter	Use	Material
Foley two-way	Short term	Latex/Teflon coated
Foley three-way	Irrigation system	Latex/Teflon coated
Biocath	Long term	Hydrogel coated
Folatex	Haematuria	Latex/Teflon coated

I.V. Sets

These sets are used to administer I.V. fluids. They are sterile, pyrogen free, disposable, relatively inexpensive and simple to use. The main disadvantage is lack of accuracy. Methods other than gravity must be used when accuracy is required in TPN or Paediatric therapy.

Components of I.V. Set

(i) A plastic spike: To pierce the rubber closure or plastic seal on the I.V. container.

(ii) A drip chamber: For trapping the air and adjusting the flow rate with clamp.

(iii) Clamp: Adjustable clamp of screw or roller type pinches the tubing to regulate the flow.

(iv) A polyvinyl chloride tubing terminating in gum-rubber injection port.

The flow rate should be accurate to ensure patient safety and optimum drug efficacy. Inaccurate flow rate can cause:

(i) Phlebitis or thrombophlebitis.

(ii) Delayed or toxic response to drug therapy.

(iii) Metabolic problems and speed shock.

(iv) Pulmonary oedema resulting in impaired cardiac and renal functions.

Hence it is an important function of I.V. therapist to maintain constant accurate flow rate. Infusion pumps are the electromechanical devices designed to automatically control the intravenous infusion. Four types of devices are available viz. Gravity feed controllers, drip-rate pumps, volumetric pumps and syringe drivers.

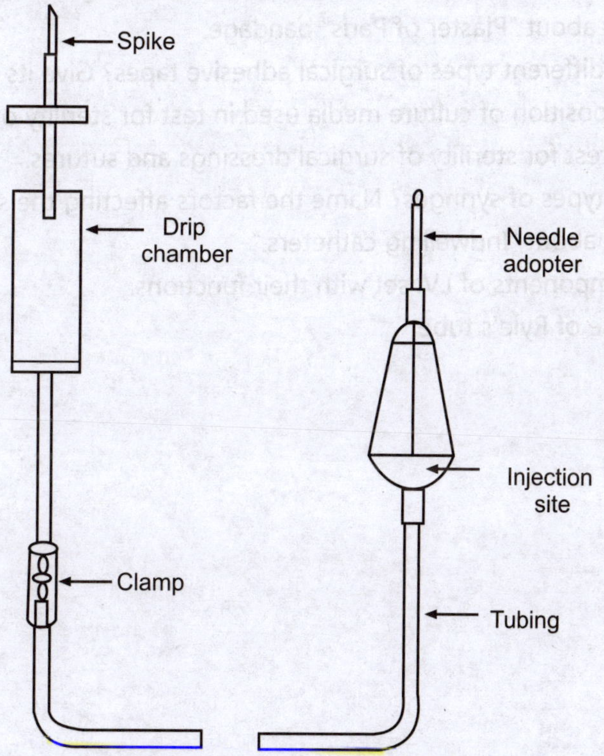

Fig. 12.1: Administration Set

Ryle's Tube: A tube of narrow calibre and short length is used for stomach wash especially in case of children. A number 8 to 12 French rubber catheter is used. About 25 cm length is necessary to reach the stomach. This distance should be marked with a piece of adhesive tape. The catheter is passed through nose or mouth in the stomach. After reaching the stomach a 20 or 50 ml glass syringe is attached to the upper end of the catheter and the stomach contents aspirated. The antidote solution is then introduced in small volumes.

Sterilization: The glass syringes are sterilized by dry heat in oven whereas plastics (catheters, Ryle's tube) and rubber material are sterilised by autoclaving or ethylene oxide.

QUESTIONS

1. Give the ideal properties of surgical dressing.
2. What are the different tests used for evaluating the quality of surgical cotton?
3. Describe the labelling conditions for gauze.
4. Give the uses of absorbent ribbon gauze.
5. Classify bandages with examples.
6. Describe the support and compression bandages.
7. Give the composition of paste used in medicated bandage.
8. Write in short about "Plaster of Paris" bandage.
9. What are the different types of surgical adhesive tapes? Give its uses.
10. Give the composition of culture media used in test for sterility of surgical dressings.
11. Describe the test for sterility of surgical dressings and sutures.
12. What are the types of syringes? Name the factors affecting the selection of syringe.
13. Write in short about "Indwelling catheters."
14. Name the components of I.V. set with their functions.
15. Explain the use of Ryle's tube.

***

13

COMPUTERS IN PHARMACY

Introduction

Prior to the study of computer applications in Pharmacy, we must understand the elements of a computer system which are listed below:

1. **Central Processing Unit (CPU):** It is the heart of the computer system. It performs calculations, executes program instructions and manages the flow of data. The CPU is the core of the computer's hardware.

2. **Software:** These are the programs (set of instructions) used to tell the CPU what to do with the data it has. Various software programs are available such as word processing, spreadsheets, keeping account records and various statistical analysis. Many software programs are predesigned or specially written to meet the specific needs of pharmacies or for use in a hospital.

3. **Memory:** Two types of memories are present in the CPU.

(i) **ROM:** Read Only Memory. It can be read but not erased when the computer is turned off.

(ii) **RAM:** Random Access Memory. When the computer is turned off, the RAM is erased. The amount of RAM determines how much information or calculations the computer can work with at a time. Normally at least 512 K of RAM (1K = 1000 bytes) is desired where 1 byte = single letter, nurnber or symbol. If the computer has a RAM less than this, it may not work with some of the software available.

4. **Storage:** The computer has two drives for the storage of data viz. disk drives and hard drives. The disk drives are attached to the CPU so that the external information can be transmitted to the internal processing system, from which it is sent to the diskettes for storage in the form of files. The hard drives are directly linked to the processing unit and installed within the internal operating system. Hence it can store and retrieve the data more rapidly than disk drives.

5. **Key Board and Monitor:** These are equipments used to run the computer. The keyboard is similar to that of typewriter with some additional keys. The monitor or cathod ray tube (CRT) is the screen which may be either colour or monochrome.

6. **Printer:** It is an electronic device which prints information based on the commands given to it by CPU.

Computer Applications in Hospital

Computers have played an important role in the development of clinical pharmacy practice and basic pharmacy research. The use of computers in hospital administration and medical research becomes the need of large hospitals. The computer is a processor which processes large quantity of data which may be numbers, letters or picture elements very fastly and accurately.

The modern physician is so busy that he does not have enough time to give personal attention to the patients. Todays pharmacist's responsibilities are also increased. Following is a list of common capabilities and functions of modern hospital computer system.

1. Patient record database management.
2. Entries of medication orders.
3. Preparation of lists.
4. Patient medication profile.
5. Drug use review.
6. Drug therapy monitoring and problem detection.
7. Purchasing and inventory control.
8. Billing procedures.
9. Drug formulary search and update.
10. Management information systems and decision support.
11. Integration with other hospital departments.

1. Patient Record Data Base Management

A pharmacy computer system must manage that the pharmacy's patient record database is continually updated to reflect the current status of all patients. Updated is done by assessing the database of admitting department to determine the information about recent admissions, discharges and patient transfers (ADT). The computer system should be capable of producing the other information such as:

Present diagnosis, allergies, weight, height, name of attending physician and other special notes regarding the patient.

2. Entries of Medication Orders

Rapid processing of drug orders is the essential function of computer system. Formatted data entry screens should allow easy entry and retrieval of orders. A pharmacist should be able to retrieve orders for review prior to administration to patient. Data may be entered by use of codes for drug name, dosing schedule. All the drug orders should contain the following:

Drug name (code)
Drug generic name and strength
Route of administration
Dosage schedule
Starting data
Stopping date
Physician code
Pharmacist verification code.

Features: The system should be capable of rapidly collecting and displaying entries by patient name or room number. It should be capable of scheduling, starting and stopping date automatically and separating the orders of patients on active drug therapy from those with no drug therapy.

3. Preparation of Lists

The computer system should be capable of producing the labels and reports in the form of:

(i) Patient medication profile

(ii) "Fill-lists" for preparation of individual doses

(iii) List of medications charged

(iv) Drug order renewal lists for the prescriber and

(v) Medication administration record (MARV.

Orders entered for IV solutions, admixtures and total parenteral nutrition (TPN) should be separately prepared. These orders should contain the following information.

"Patient" and "Medication Order" identifying information Start date and Stop date.

Administration rate and Order status (conditional or active).

The system should be capable of calculating the flow rates and checking the incompatibilities. It should allow the conditional entry and its checking by pharmacist. The system should be able to prepare the lists of solutions soon to expire and to be prepared at pharmacy.

4. Patient Medication Profile

A pharmacist keeps prescription records of patients which are referred to as patient medication profile. The purpose of patient medication profile is to provide the history of patient's previous medication including a note on any idiosyncracies, allergies and untoward medication effects together with a record of his current, medication. This enables the patient's medication to be monitored and provides the data for consultation. The patient's medication profile contains the following basic information:

Patient's name	:	....
Address	:	....
Telephone No.	:	....
Age	:	....
Date of birth	:	....
Allergy or Sensitivities	:	....
Special diet	:	....
Chronic Medical Conditions	:	....
Date of Prescription Dispensed	:	....
Prescription item	:	....
Dosage instruction	:	....
Quantity	:	....
Repeats (if any) and Prescriber	:	....

<table>
<tr><td colspan="4">Mr.
Mrs.
Miss.
Master Surname</td><td colspan="2">First name</td><td colspan="2">Home address</td></tr>
<tr><td colspan="2">Tel: Home:
Business:</td><td colspan="2">Date of
Birth</td><td colspan="2"></td><td colspan="2"></td></tr>
<tr><td colspan="2">Medical Practitioner
Tel:</td><td colspan="2"></td><td colspan="2">Known
Sensitivity</td><td colspan="2">Business Address
Self/Husband</td></tr>
<tr><th>Date</th><th>Prescription No.</th><th>Medication</th><th>Dose</th><th>Quantity</th><th>No. of Rept.</th><th>Prescriber</th><th>Price
₹ Ps.</th></tr>
<tr><td></td><td></td><td></td><td></td><td></td><td></td><td></td><td></td></tr>
</table>

Patient's Medication Profile

Medication Administration Records (MAR)

The practice of keeping complete medication records is more useful and beneficial to all the health professionals in the hospital. The computerization in a hospital for this purpose is must for the following reasons:

1. Preventing the consumption of more time, personnel and money.
2. It acts as a guide to prescribe the drugs. Since the records of patient medication profiles are computerised and maintained, the physician considers the same while prescribing the drugs.
3. Computerization avoids drug-drug interactions and adverse effects of the drugs.
4. It is also useful for assessing and evaluating the economical position of the hospital and helps in maintaining the same.
5. It also helps Pharmacists in extending their professional expertise to physicians and advising doctors on medicines and counselling patients.

5. Drug Use Review (DUR)

Drug use review can be defined as procedure for reviewing, analysing and improving the quality of prescribing drugs and advising their use in medical practice.

The drug use review in hospitals are generally drug specific or drug category specific. The common drug use reviews in the hospital are monitoring the usage of:

(i) Drugs with high unit cost.

(ii) Drugs added to the formulary on conditional basis.

(iii) Restricted drugs.

The computer system should be capable of producing the DUR reports according to different parameters such as physician, date, combinations of patients, age, sex, weight, associated diseases. The DUR report may either be aggregate usage report or detailed report.

6. Medication Monitoring (Drug Therapy Monitoring)

The computerised medication monitoring systems have been used to give a warning of potential adverse drug reactions. Information from many area is gathered to form a broad patient data base. The system integrates the gathered information and returns warning messages and suggestions regarding patient drug therapy to the pharmacist. The program 'HELP' (Health Evaluation through Logical Processing) is used to allow experts in a medical speciality for defining the criteria of medical decision-making. The broad base and flexibility of HELP permits complete drug monitoring. After receiving the warning message from the computer, the pharmacist contacts the doctor or nursing staff and discuss the situation. The system can be used to produce prescription labels and patient drug profiles. This system makes the pharmacist more efficient and accurate in monitoring patient drug therapy. The system issues warnings more quickly than manual monitoring methods.

Daily updated copies of drug profiles for each patient helps the pharmacist in reviewing the patient drug therapy. The drug profiles together with various drug interaction (drug-drug, drug-laboratory agent, drug-allergy, drug-disease) detection capabilities of the computer greatly enhances the pharmacist's service contribution.

Features of the System

1. The messages are presented in the form of pharmacological summary.
2. The drug interaction messages are integrated with computerized drug profile system.
3. All drug interactions which could occur in the patient's current drug therapy is reported by this system.
4. The information received from the system is used by either a physician or a pharmacist in the clinical area.
5. The system is useful in reducing the drug interaction and beneficial to interns and medical students.

The another system called "MEDIPHER" (monitoring and evaluation of drug interaction by a pharmacy oriented reporting system) can also be used for monitoring the drug interactions. This system issues the warnings when potentially interacting drugs are prescribed for a patient.

Data base: If the prescription containing many drugs is entered in the computer for billing purpose, immediately the computer scans the drugs and issues the warning if there is possibility of drug interaction. Thus, the computer helps in avoiding the drug interactions.

The computer also issues warning, if two or more brands of same drug are entered in it. Thus it avoids a drug duplication.

If two or more drugs of same class are included in the prescription that can be detected by the computer, a warning is issued, if the program of drug class duplication screening is included in the computer.

Whenever the pharmacist is very busy, he may pass on his work of displaying the contents and instructions of medication and label printing to the computer after entering the prescription. This is useful in avoiding the human errors.

7. Purchasing and Inventory Control

A computer can be effectively used for purchasing and inventory control in a hospital pharmacy as follows:

(a) Maintenance of perpectual Inventory Control: Whenever an item is added to stock or removed from stock, immediately the position of stock can be updated by the computer. This operation of the computer is intimately linked to other operations such as receipt of good, dispensing of goods, billing of goods, return of goods etc.

(b) Maintaining the Inventory Records: For annual auditing of the pharmacy department, records of numerous items are required to be typed laboriously. This can be overcome by use of computer through perpectual inventory control and these records can be made ready for inspection at any time when needed.

(c) Calculation of Inventory: The computer can be used for calculating the value of each item recorded and these values can be printed out. The A, B, C analysis of items recorded can be done on the basis of their volume and cost.

(d) Automatic Updating of Price: The computer can be effectively used whenever there are changes in the prices of items recorded.

(e) Evaluation of Demand: The requirement of any item in the pharmacy can be assessed by analysing the movement of various items from stock within a period of one year.

8. Billing Procedures

The patient billing is a time consuming but important activity for the hospital pharmacy and its accounting department. The hospitals accounting department is the first typical area where computerization is needed. The pharmacy department must assure that all drugs leaving the pharmacy are billed to the appropriate patient's account. The computer system automatically charges the patient for all medications and I.V. solutions ordered. Other drugs charges may be entered in the computer manually.

The billing system should be such that it automatically accesses the fee schedule for items billed and is capable of making the changes in fee structure easily. The information usually included in the bill is:

Name, account number and address, Type of drug services received, charge and date.

9. Formulary Search and Update

The record of approved formulary drugs is maintained in a file. The computer system should be capable of displaying all drugs by descriptors code, therapeutic category or generic name.

10. Management Information System

It is most important and essential to develop and maintain an information system which will help the management in decision-making.

11. Integration with Other departments of the Hospital

While designing and implementing the computer system for pharmacy; its dependence with other departments of the hospital must be considered. These departments are purchasing or accounting, billing, admitting, nursing patient care units, dietary and laboratory.

Drug Information Retrieval and Storage

Computerization of narcotics and other controlled substances may help in preventing excessive supplies and unauthorised dispensing of such drugs. The specific identification codes for the drugs are given to authorized person. The drug control authorities are directly linked through computers to such records and are able to trace quickly the erring employees. The program used for this purpose is DAWN (Drug Abuse Warning Network).

Another program called "CLAUDE" (Computerised Listing of Abnormal and Unusual Drug Effects) containing 17,500 abnormal effects on laboratory test of 1,500 drugs may be computerised to match the laboratory test effects of drugs with patient. Because scanning manually for every patient is time consuming. Computer matches it quickly and prints the warning about the results of laboratory tests.

Computerization is must in the area of drug information. The new technology 'Data base' is now developed to convert printed information to computerized' information. These data bases could be online and can be contacted through telephone lines. Martindale's extra pharmacopoeia is available on-line.

Some other data bases available on-line are:

(i) MEDLARS (Medical Literature Analysis and Retrieval System).

The earliest effort to computerize medical information retrieval resulted in the creation of MEDLARS by NLM.

(ii) MEDLINE (MEDLARS ON-LINE)

(iii) NLM (National Library of Medicine)

(iv) MICROMEDEX: It is a microcomputer based retrieval system that uses a laser disk at the site for storage of data.

(v) International Pharmaceutical Abstracts (I.P.A.): It is available in an on-line print version.

(vi) Pharmaceutical News Index (PNI) contains current news about devices, cosmetics and related health industries. It provides newsletters which are not covered by printing in abstracts and indexes. It is updated weekly.

Advantages: The most important advantage is time saving in conducting literature searches. A pharmacist may require several hours to research a particular therapeutic question from a literature search covering about 10 years of articles. It can be done in minutes and the computer search is more pleasant.

Only few seconds are required to broaden a computer search from a specific drug to entire therapeutic class, but manually it is a tedious job to search in the 'INDEX MEDICUS'.

Retrospective searching can be carried out efficiently.

Computer applications in retail pharmacy (Community Pharmacy):

Computers have invaded every walk of life and almost all commercial organisation and business firms have undergone significant computerization with no exception of community pharmacy establishments. At present community pharmacies use computers for selected pharmaceutical functions. While there are many possible uses; the systems are not now fully developed and utilized. Following is a list of majority of community pharmacy functions that could be computerized.

1. **Clerical:** Preparation of prescription labels.

   Providing a receipt for patient. Generation of hard copy record of transactions. Calculation of total prescription cost. Maintenance of perpetual record of inventory status. Accumulation of suggested orders based on suggested order quantities. Automatically order required inventory via electronic transmission. Calculation and storing of payrolls. Preparation of annual withholding statements.

2. **Managerial:** Preparation of daily sales report.

   Generation of complete sales analysis as required for a day, week, month, year and to date for number of prescriptions handled and amounts in cash. Estimation of profit and financial ratio analysis. Production of drug usage reports. Calculation of gross margins, reported in all manner of details. Calculate number of prescriptions handled per unit time, to help in staff scheduling. Printing of billing and payment summaries.

3. **Professional:** Building a patient profile.

   Storing of information on drug and other allergies to warn about possible problems.

   Retrieval of current drug regiment for review. Monitoring of drug utilization. Updating of patient information in file. Printing of warnings of drug-drug and drug-food interactions. Maintaining of physicians files including speciality, designation address, phone, office hours etc.

QUESTIONS

---

1. How does the computer aids the clinical pharmaceutical services of the hospital ?
2. Explain the importance of computer in the inventory control in hospital.
3. Write a note on "Medication monitoring".
4. Describe the use of computer in maintenance of records.
5. Name the various data bases.
6. Describe the followings:
   (a) DUR
   (b) Patient medication profile
   (c) Drug information retrieval and storage systems.
7. Explain the applications of computer in community pharmacy.

***

Part II - Clinical Pharmacy

1

INTRODUCTION TO CLINICAL PHARMACY PRACTICE

In the last three decades, clinical pharmacy has come of age and the clinical pharmacist is now able to dispense knowledge as a product to patients and physicians. As new drugs were released on the market, pharmacy profession began to move towards pharmacology, clinical therapeutics and pharmacokinetics. Hospital pharmacy seemed to take the lead in this clinical movement as several studies indicated that with many powerful drugs used in hospitals adverse drug reactions were a serious problem that needed the involvement of clinical pharmacy services.

Baker (1976) has defined clinical pharmacy as pharmacist involvement in monitoring patient therapy and giving advice which directly influences the decisions about drug therapy and the way in which it is administered.

Educationally, clinical pharmacy may be defined as a concept which considers the treatment and care of patients by members of the health team in the presence of pharmacy students, with particular emphasis on the safe and appropriate use of drugs.

Objectives: The clinical pharmacy program is setup with the aim of providing the student pharmacist with an educational experience in clinical setting. The program is designed to help the student better prepare for his future role as a health professional. The objectives of clinical pharmacy are as follows:

The program gives an opportunity to the student to develop himself for using his independent judgement by following a drug therapy of selected patients and through case presentation technique.

- It gives the student experience in small group presentations and in answering questions regarding therapy asked by his professional colleagues and physicians and/or nurses.
- It also gives an opportunity to the student to observe and interact with physician to get a better understanding of current medical practice.
- It gives an opportunity to students to work with paramedical personnel and increase his knowledge about their attitudes and contributions to patient care,
- It helps the student to learn a patient orientation towards drug therapy so that he can provide better professional services to his patients.
- It gives the student a better knowledge of the effects of drugs on diagnostic tests and various drug interactions which may occur in multiple drug therapy so that he is able to give a better service to his patients.
- It gives the student an experience about the drug information retrieval through drug evaluation.
- It also gives the student an experience of institutional environment by recognizing that most pharmacists practice in an institution.

Clinical Pharmacy Services of Pharmacist

The following is a list of Pharmacist's Services:

1. Compounds and dispenses prescription.
2. Prepares medication histories for the patient's permanent medical record.
3. Assumes care and responsibility for distribution of controlled substances.
4. Explains the directions for use of prescription medicines at the time of delivery of prescriptions to ambulatory patients.
5. Helps in selecting and monitoring drug therapy.
6. Patient education and counselling.
7. Establishes and monitors a system to insure proper storage of pharmacy items such as insulin and other biological products.
8. Selects the manufacturing source of drug products to be purchased under generic names.
9. Maintains prescription profile records for ambulatory patients.

10. Participates in the management of medical emergencies, adverse drug reactions and acute and chronic disease states.
11. Develops guidelines for the use of antibiotics.
12. Detects and reports the adverse drug reactions.
13. Participates in drug use reviews and quality assurance programs.
14. Applies pharmacokinetic principles in determining or modifying the dose of selected drugs.
15. Provides formal and informal consultations with physicians regarding patient drug therapy problems.
16. Initiates and participates in research including clinical drug investigations.

In addition to providing the above services pharmacists have a responsibility to communicate advances in development and delivery of clinical pharmacy services to the health care community through appropriate publications, presentations and programs.

The following diagram illustrates the role of clinical pharmacist in various areas of making decisions on drug therapy.

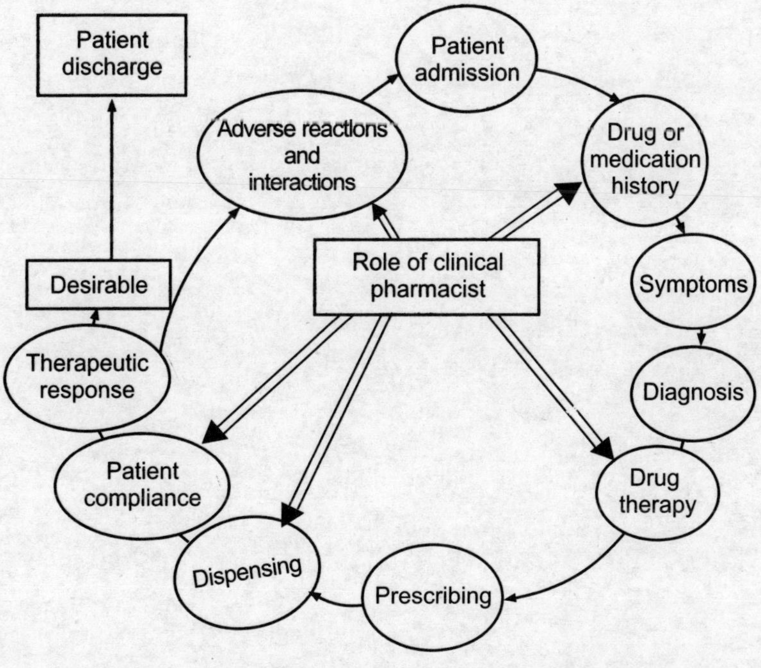

Fig. 1.1

QUESTIONS

1. Define "Clinical Pharmacy". Give the reason for the involvement of clinical pharmacy.
2. What are the objectives of clinical pharmacy ?
3. Give the functions of a clinical pharmacist.
4. What is the role of a clinical pharmacist in various areas of making decisions on drug therapy ?

***

2

MODERN DISPENSING ASPECTS

The goals of therapy are not achieved unless the patient understands and follows the instructions for use of drugs prescribed. The pharmacist is the logical health professional to assume the major responsibility in minimising noncompliance. Of priority importance is the need to strengthen communications with patient and physician.

Role of Pharmacist

For safe and effective drug therapy patients need to be well informed about medications and their use. Knowledgeable patients exhibit increased compliance with drug regimens, resulting in improved therapeutic outcomes. Therefore, it is the responsibility of the pharmacist and other health professionals to inform the patients, properly about their drug therapy.

Patient Counseling

By using various techniques of communications (verbal, written or audio-visual) the pharmacist should inform, educate and counsel patients about the following items for each drug:

1. Name of drug (Different names with synonyms).
2. Use of drug and its action.
3. Route of administration and dosage schedule; dosage form and time of administration.
4. Directions for preparations.
5. Directions and precautions for administration.
6. Common side effects of the drug.
7. Self-monitoring of drug therapy.
8. Adequate storage of the drugs.
9. Contraindications and interactions of the drug.
10. Information about prescription refill.
11. What to do in the event of missed dose (s).
12. Specific information to specific patients regarding certain drugs.

A patient needs practical, useful information and the pharmacist should share his knowledge and to the patient communicate the above information.

1. **Name of the Drug and its Action:** The pharmacist should inform the patient not only the name of the drug but also its other names (Synonyms). He must explain the use of that drug and action on the body. In brief he has to explain how the drug acts?

2. **Route of administration:** It is important for the pharmacist to inform the patient about the route of administration of drug. Whether the drug is to be taken orally or it is to be applied locally or to be used in the eye, ear or nose or inserted rectally or vaginally.

The pharmacist should be sure that the patient understands how to use ophthalmic preparations, and suppositories. Cocoa butter suppositories should be gently rubbed with fingers to melt the surface so that it achieves lubrication and ease in administration. In case of eye drops, it can easily be demonstrated to the patient by placing the finger below the lower eyelid and pulling down and installation.

3. **Time of administration:** The pharmacist should instruct the patient when to take the medication e.g. some drugs should be taken on empty stomach i.e. about 1 hour before meal 2-3 hours after meal to insure adequate absorption of the drug. The patient should be provided with a medication calender (which contains clock hours in vertical column indicating the name of drug and dosage to be taken at that time, the horizontal column contains the days of the month from 1-31) to avoid the duplication of the dosage.

4. **Duration of therapy:** The pharmacist should encourage the patient to continue taking the medicine for the prescribed duration of the treatment. He should explain (specially in case of antibiotic therapy) that the course of treatment must be completed to achieve the best results.

5. **Storage of drugs:** The pharmacist should instruct the patient regarding the storage of drugs, though these are labelled on the container. The patient should be advised to store the drugs in a separate cabinet where children cannot reach.

6. **Adverse effects of drug:** The patient should be informed about the adverse effects of the drug, but it is not necessary to inform about all the side effects e.g. Headache. If informed about headache, the patient may induce headache due to suggestion or it may scare the patient into not taking the medicine. The patient should be informed of those side effects which will allay his fears and help him to avoid injury to himself e.g. change in colour of urine drowsiness.

7. **Restrictions:** The patient should be well informed regarding foods and drugs he should avoid during the therapy.

E.g.: (1) Restriction of tyramine containing foods in patients on MAO inhibitor therapy.

(2) Restriction of aspirin in patients on anticoagulant therapy.

8. **Allergic reactions:** Before dispensing the drugs like penicillin or sulphonamides (having higher incidence of allergic reaction), the pharmacist should ask the patient about his allergic reactions in the past. It helps in avoiding the further complications during treatment.

9. **Removal of drug from package:** The patient is not familiar with the packaging of the product, as the pharmacist. Hence, the pharmacist should demonstrate the method of removal of drug from package to the patient so that he can handle it properly.

10. Refill information: The pharmacist should inform the patient verbally, whether the prescription is refillable or not. If it is, then for how many times it may be refilled and length of time during which it may be refilled. If it is non-refillable, he should be informed, so that he can contact the physician for the same drug if needed.

Patient Compliance

Patient compliance is defined as the patient's understanding and adherence to the directions for use of prescribed drugs.

"Patient non-compliance" means the patient is not following the directions for use of prescribed drugs. He is at fault for inappropriate use of medication. Many times the noncompliance is due to two reasons.

(i) Adequate instructions are not provided to the patient by pharmacist or physician, and

(ii) Instructions are not presented in a manner that patient understands.

It is a major problem in ambulatory patients and in children.

Consequences of Non-compliances:

The patient non-compliance results in either underutilization of drug or overutilization of drug.

Effects of Underutilization of Drug

It may happen due to the following reasons:

1. Taking less than the prescribed dose.
2. Discontinuing the drug before completing the course.
3. Omiting one or more doses.

Underutilization may result in:

(a) Risk of toxicity: If the physician is unaware of the patient's non-compliance, the physician may increase the frequency of doses or prescribe a more potent antihypertensive drugs, which could result in toxicity e.g. in the treatment of hypertensive patient.

(b) Danger of death: One report of anticonvulsant drugs reveals that underutilization of anticonvulsant drug results in uncontrollable seizures and death.

(c) In patients with C.C.F., digoxin and hydrochlorthiazide are used together. Potassium chloride is also administered to these patients to replace potassium. (Potassium loss occurs due to diuretic action). If patient stop taking potassium chloride, the potassium depletion results, making the heart more sensitive to digoxin and toxicity of cardiac glycosides occur.

(d) In treatment of infectious disease with antibiotic therapy the patient may stop taking the drug when the symptoms disappear and hence he will not use all the prescribed medication. This results in recurrence of the infection. e.g. Tuberculosis.

(e) Omitting a single dose of contraceptive pill may result in an unwanted pregnancy.

Effects of Overutilization of Drug

It may happen due to the following reasons:

(i) Taking more than the prescribed dose.

(ii) Taking more than the prescribed number of doses.

(iii) Taking a dose at a time other than when needed.

(iv) Taking the same medication from two or more different bottles simultaneously.

Overutilization of drug results in an increased risk of adverse reactions and toxicity. The problem of drug abuse results from excessive use of medications.

Factors Contributing to Non-compliance

Following are the various factors that result in patient non-compliance:

- Poor understanding of instructions.
- Unpleasant taste of medication.
- Fear of becoming drug dependent.
- Side effects of the drug.
- Multiple drug therapy.
- Asymptomatic nature of the patient.
- Delay of physician or pharmacist resulting in bored waiting for the drug.
- Measurement of medication.
- Cost of medication.
- Frequency of administration.
- Duration of therapy
- Illness.

Poor Understanding of Instructions: The instructions given by the physician or pharmacist may not be followed correctly. There may be wrong interpretation of the instructions given on the label e.g. in interpreting a prescription that read "Tetracycline 250 mg every 6 hours." Some patients interpret it as around the clock (24 hrs.) and take the dose 4 times while some take it as to 18 hours (awaking duration) and take the dose only 3 times.

Unpleasant taste of medication: It is common problem with the use of oral liquids in children. Use of flavours and sweeteners in antimicrobial agents help to improve the compliance.

Fear of becoming drug dependent: Some patients think that they may become drug dependent for activities like sleep.

Side effects: The adverse effects (nausea, vomitting, hair loss) drugs are sufficiently, due reduction in quality of life which results in noncompliance.

The ability of certain antipsychotic drugs and an antihypertensives to cause sexual dysfunction have also resulted in non-compliance.

The warning of possible adverse reactions to the patient may result in non-compliance.

Multiple drug therapy: It is generally felt that the greater the number of drugs a patient is taking the higher is the risk of non-compliance. The similarity of appearance (size, colour, shape) of certain drugs may result in confusion and thus non-compliance. e.g. The patient may get confused between two small white tablets one of 0.25 mg digoxin and another of 40 mg furosemide.

Asymptomatic nature of patient: In cage of an asymptomatic patient, it is difficult to convince patient by explaining the value of drug therapy. This results in non-compliance especially in hypertensive patients, especially as the patient remains asymptomatic even after discontinuing therapy.

Delay of physician or pharmacist visit: If a patient has to wait for a long time in getting the prescription or drugs from physician or pharmacist, the poorer is the compliance. Reduction in these delays have resulted in more favourable patient response.

Measurement of medication: Many times a patient gets confused in measuring the medication especially liquid preparation or number of tablets.

Cost of medication: The expenses involved is a major reason for some patients for not having the drugs or some patients take the medication less frequently than required. As soon as the symptoms disappear, the patient may discontinue the higher priced drugs such as antibiotics.

Frequency of administration: Many drugs must be given at frequent intervals to maintain the specific blood level. Due to frequent administration of the drugs the patient's routine life gets distributed resulting in non-compliance. Hence, the dosage regimen should be simple and convenient.

Duration of therapy: There is greater risk of non-compliance in patients having chronic disorders requiring longer duration of therapy.

Illness: The nature of patient's illness may contribute to non-compliance. Patients with chronic hypertension, psychiatric disorders and schizophrenia are more likely to be non-complaint.

Steps to Improve Compliance

1. Identification of risk factors that may contribute to non-compliance.
2. Educating the patient: By means of effective verbal and written communication with the patient.
3. Development of treatment plan with recognition of patient's normal pattern of activities.
4. Designation of specific times of day at which medication is to be taken.
5. Monitoring therapy.
6. Patient motivation.

Advice for Use of Common Drugs

The effective communication between pharmacist and patient greatly reduces the non-compliance. Advice to patients on their medication must also be based on knowledge of the action of the drug. The following type of advice or information is required by patient on their prescribed medicines.

1. Indications.
2. Dose to be taken.
3. Frequency of dosing. Specifications about timing.
4. Administration in relation to food.
5. How to use special administration devices.
6. What to do if dose is missed.
7. Adverse effects
   (a) Its recognition and
   (b) Action to be taken
8. Duration of therapy
9. Prevention of the followings:
   Alcohol, oral contraceptive, driving, specific hobbies.

Examples of few drugs for :vhich specific and simple advice is required, are listed below:

1. **Antidiabetic drug:** Do not drink alcoholic beverages.
2. **Antacid tablet:** Do not swallow but chew it.
3. **MAO inhibitors:** Avoid cheese, alcoholic beverages, and liver or yeast extract.
4. **Salicylates, phenyl butazone and oxyphen butazone:** Do not take on empty stomach.
5. **Liquid Paraffin:** Do not use for prolonged time.
6. **Diazepam:** Drug causes drowsiness hence do not drive a vehicle or work on dangerous machinery.
7. **Ampicillin:** (1) It should be taken on empty stomach i.e. one hour before or two hours after food. (2) Complete the course of treatment otherwise recurrence on infection takes place.
8. **Spermicidal jellies and creams:** These should be. applied 10-30 minutes before intercourse and must remain in the vagina for 6-8 hours afterward.
9. **Phenolphthalein (laxative):** It may colour the faeces and urine pink.
10. **Bisacodyl, tetracycline:** Do not take with milk or antacid.
11. **Cascara sagrada:** Avoid breast feeding. It may colour the urine pale yellow to reddish brown.
12. **Aluminium hydroxide:** Constipation may occur.
13. **Phenytoin, phenobarbital:** Expose yourself to sunlight in the morning.
14. **Diphenhydramine:** It may cause sedation.

15. Nitrates: (1) After long term use, do not suddenly stop using it. Stopping suddenly may bring on: (1) attacks of angina. (2) Dizziness, light headedness or a fainting feeling may occur especially when you get up quickly from lying or sitting position.

16. Penicillins: (1) If diarrhoea occurs, do not take any antidiarrhoeal medicine. (2) Oral contraceptives are ineffective during ampicillin or penicillin – V therapy.

General Advice About How to Store the Medicine

- ❑ Store away from heat and direct sunlight.
- ❑ Keep out of reach of children.
- ❑ Do not store medicines in the refrigerator unless directed to do so.
- ❑ Do not keep outdated medicine or medicine no longer needed.

Medication History

It is the pharmacist's responsibility to obtain and document the medication history for ambulatory patients, by interviewing them. The history includes the past and present use of prescription and non-prescription drugs, drug allergies, previous adverse effects associated with medication use and an estimate of the patient's compliance with medication regimen.

The initial drug history should be completed within 24-48 hours after admission. The standard form for reporting the findings of initial drug history is given below:

PATIENT DRUG HISTORY			
Date	Note progress, complications, consultations, changes in diagnosis, condition on discharge, instructions to patient.		
	Allergies and Adverse effects		
	Prescription drugs	**Start**	**Stop**
	Non-prescription drugs (Used regularly)	Yes	No
	(Use "✓" mark)	–	–
	Alcohol	–	–
	Caffeine	–	–
	Tobacco	–	–
	Analgesics	–	–
	Antacids	–	–
	Laxatives	–	–
	Sedatives	–	–
	Diet preparations	–	–
	Skin products	–	–
	Haemarrhoidal preparations	–	–
	Other	–	–
	Comments:	–	–

Objectives of Medication History

1. To find out which drug causes allergy and adverse drug reactions.
2. To prepare a list of patient's current and past medications.
3. To study the patient's compliance for drugs.
4. To know the patient's self prescribing habit and which OTC drugs he prefers to take.
5. To study his routine life i.e. various habits, such as alcohol, tea, tobacco etc.
6. To know about the diet preparations of the patient.

QUESTIONS

1. Describe the role of pharmacist in patient counselling.
2. Define patient "Compliance" and give the reasons for non-compliance.
3. Describe the consequences of patient non-compliance.
4. Name the factors contributing to non-compliance. Describe any three.
5. How will you improve the patient compliance?
6. What advice will you give about following drugs:
   (i) Diazepam
   (ii) Ampicillin
   (iii) Antacid tablet
   (iv) MAO inhibitors
   (v) Salicylates.
7. Write in short about medication history.

***

3

MEDICAL TERMINOLOGY

The aim of this chapter is to help students to acquire a good knowledge of medical terms in current use in practice of medicine.

Medicine: It is a term denoting all aspects in the science of the prevention, investigation and treatment of disease.

Disease: It is a condition in which some abnormality of structure or function, or of both structure and function, is present in some part or parts of the body.

The word disease is synonymous with other terms, when used in the right context, such as disorder, ailment, pathological condition, illness, sickness, morbidity or morbid condition.

Some general terms may be used while describing the different forms of disease as given below:

Descriptive term	Meaning
Acute	Rapid onset and progress of disease.
Chronic	Slow onset and progress of disease.
Organic	Associated with abnormality in structure of organ.
Congenital	Present at birth.
Acquired	Acquired after birth.
Familial	Occurring in families.
Functional	Associated with abnormality of function.
Systemic	Involving the body system.
Local	Involving only a part of the body.

Types of Diseases and Their Causes

- **Congenital**
  - (i) Genetic factor e.g. *Haemophilia.*
  - (ii) Environmental factors e.g. *Congenital syphilis from maternal infections.*
  - (iii) Combined genetic and environmental factors: e.g. *Congenital heart disease, congenital pyloric stenosis.*
- **Traumatic:** Occurs due to:
  - (i) Violence: e.g. *Fracture, dislocation.*
  - (ii) Mechanical irritation: e.g. *Bedsores.*
  - (iii) External physical agents. e.g. *Thermal burns.*
  - (iv) External chemical agents e.g. *Acid burns.*

- **Neoplastic:** Due to formation of tumours.
- **Infective:** Due to infection of pathogenic microbes e.g. *Influenza, tuberculosis.*
- **Poisoning by Chemicals:** e.g. *Arsenic poisoning.*
- **Allergic:** Due to hypersensitivity e.g. *Hay fever.*
- **Endocrine:** Due to disorders in endocrine glands.
- **Psychiatric:** Due to abnormal conditions of mind.
- **Iatrogenic:** Due to treatment given for other diseases e.g. *Drug induced diseases.*
- **Metabolic:** Due to disturbed metabolism e.g. *Gout.*
- **Idiopathic:** Due to unknown cause.

Some important classes of drugs used in the practice of medicine are listed below:

- **Adrenergic:** Drug which mimic the response obtained by stimulation of sympathetic or adrenergic nerves. These are also called as *Sympathomimetics.*
- **Adrenergic blocking agents:** Drugs which block the effects of adrenergic system. Also called as sympatholytics or adrenolytics.
- **Alkylating agents:** Disrupt the process of cell division by affecting DNA in nucleus, by addition of alkyl groups. Used as cytotoxic drugs in neoplastic disorders.
- **Allergy:** Any abnormal or altered reaction to an antigen or allergen. It is used to indicate the hypersensitivity of body cells to specific substance.
- **Anaesthetic:** A drug that produces general anaesthesia i.e. loss of sensation with reversible loss of consciousness.
- **Analeptics:** Drugs which stimulate CNS.
- **Analgesics:** Drugs which relieve pain.
- **Antacids:** An agent that reduces or neutralises the acidity of the gastric juice or any other secretion.
- **Antibiotics:** Substances produced by living organisms which can destroy or prevent growth and multiplication of various pathogenic microbes.
- **Anticoagulants:** Drugs which reduce or prevent the coagulation of blood.
- **Anticonvulsants:** Drugs used in the treatment of epilepsy.
- **Antidote:** An agent that neutralises or counteracts the effects of poison.
- **Antidiuretics:** Drugs which decrease the output of urine.
- **Antiemetic:** Drugs which prevent emesis or vomitting.
- **Antiepileptics:** Drugs used to treat epilepsy.
- **Antifungal:** Agent preventing fungal growth.
- **Antihistamines:** Drugs used to block the action of histamine.
- **Antihypertensives:** Drugs which lower the blood pressure.
- **Antimalarials:** Drugs preventing or curing malaria.
- **Antimetabolite:** A substance that chemically resembles a particular metabolite but competes with, replaces or antagonises it.

- **Antimicrobials:** Agents that reduces, prevents or destroys pathogens.
- **Antioxidants:** A substance that inhibits oxidation.
- **Antiparasitic:** Destructive to parasites.
- **Antipyretics:** Drugs which reduce increased body temperature
- **Antirheumatic:** Preventive or curative for rheumatism.
- **Antiseptics:** Chemical substances that render disease producing micro-organisms harmless by preventing their growth and multiplication.
- **Antisialagogues:** Agents that decrease secretion of saliva.
- **Aperients:** Substances which when taken by mouth promote bowel evacuation.
- **Bitters:** The bitter principle of these drugs increase the secretion of saliva and gastric juice.
- **Carminative:** Agent that prevents the formation of gas and helps to expel it.
- **Cholagogues:** Drugs causing evacuation of gall bladder.
- **Choleretics:** Agents that increase the secretion of bile.
- **Cholinergics:** Drugs that mimic the effects of parasympathetic stimulation. Also called as para-sympathomimetics.
- **Cholinergic blocking agents:** Drugs which counteract the effects of cholinergic system. Also called as parasympatholytics or anticholinergics.
- **Disinfectants:** e.g. Chemical substances which destroy pathogenic microbes.
- **Diuretics** Drugs which enhance urine formation.
- **Hypnotics** Drugs inducing sleep resembling natural sleep.
- **Laxatives:** Drugs which loosen the bowels and facilitate the contents of bowel movements at the time of defaecation.
- **Oxytocics:** Agents which stimulate uterine contractions.
- **Purgatives:** Drugs which cause evacuation of fluid faeces.
- **Tranquillizers:** Substances which diminish anxiety and excitability by a sedative action on the nervous system.

Some Prefixes and Suffixes of the Medical Words

Prefix/Suffix	Meaning	Prefix/Suffix	Meaning
a –	absence of	homo –	same
ab –	away from	hydro –	fluid
ad –	towards	hyper –	above, excess of normal
ante –	before	hypo –	beneath, less than normal
anti –	opposed to		
auto –	self	inter –	between
baro –	pressure	intra –	within
bi –	two	iso –	same
bio –	life	– itis	inflammation
circum –	around	macro –	large

Prefix/Suffix	Meaning	Prefix/Suffix	Meaning
con –	together with	micro –	small
dys –	disordered	multi –	many
e –	out	myco –	fungus
– ectomy	cutting out, removal	– myces	fungus
		– natal	birth
epi –	upon	neo –	new
– genic	producing	– ology	science
– graphy	recording	– pathy	disease
haem –	blood	post –	after
		pre –	before
hemi –	half	Pseudo –	false
hetero –	other, differing	Sub –	below
		Supra –	above

Some Important Abbreviations used in Medical Practice

Abbreviation	Meaning	Abbreviation	Meaning
abd	Abdomen	C.V.S.	Cardiovascular system
ACTH	Adrenocorticotrophic hormone	D and C	Dilation and curettage
A/G	Albumin: Globulin Ratio	D.L.C.	Differential Leucocyte Count
AIDS	Acquired Immunity Deficiency Syndrome	D.O.A.	Dead on Arrival
A.M.	Before noon	D.U.	Duodenal Ulcer
A-V	Arteriovenous	D and V	Diarrhoea and Vomiting
AV	Atrioventricular	D.V.T.	Deep Vein Thrombosis
B.B.B.	Blood Brain Barrier	D_x	Diagnosis
	Bundle Branch Block	D.X.R.T.	Deep X-ray Therapy
B.B.T.	Basal Body Temperature	E.C.F.	Extracellular fluid
B.M.R.	Basal Metabolic Rate	E.C.G.	Electrocardiogram
B.P.	Blood Pressure	E.C.T.	Electroconvulsive therapy
	British Pharmacopoeia	E.D.D.	Expected Date of Delivery
B.U.N.	Blood Urea Nitrogen		
B.W.	Body Weight	E.E.G.	Electroencephalogram
C	Centigrade	E.M.G.	Electromyogram
$\bar{c}$	With	E.E.N.T.	Eye, Ear, Nose and Throat
cc	Cubic Centimetre		
C.C.F.	Congestive Cardiac Failure	E.O.G.,	Electro-Oculo Gram
CNS	Central Nervous System	E.O.M.	Electro-Oculo-Movements
CSF	Cerebrospinal Fluid	E.S.R.	Erythrocyte Sedimentation Rate
CT	Computerized tomography	E.S.T.	Electro Shock Therapy
CVA	Cerebro Vascular Accident	F	Fahrenheit
G.I.	Gastrointestinal	F.B.S.	Fasting Blood Sugar
gtt	Drop	F.I.D.U.	Fetal Death In Uterus
GU	Genito Urinary	F_x	Fracture
Gyn	Gynecology	G.F.R.	Glomerular Filtration Rate

Abbreviation	Meaning	Abbreviation	Meaning
H.C.V.D.	Hypertensive Cardiovascular Disease	L.A.	Left Atrium
		L.B.B.B.	Left Bundle Branch Block
Hb	Haemoglobin	L.M.P.,	Last Menstrual Period
HRT	Hormone Replacement Therapy	L.P.	Lumbar Puncture
HIV	Human Immuno Deficiency Virus	L.V.,	Left Ventricle
IBI	Intermittent Bladder Irrigation	M.C.H.	Mean Corpuscular Haemoglobin
I.C.U.	Intensive Care Unit	M.C.V.	Mean Corpuscular Volume
I.C.F.	Intracellular Fluid	M.I.	Myocardial Infarction
I.M.	Intramuscular	M.S.	Mitral Stenosis
I and O	Intake and Output		Multiple sclerosis
I.V.	Intravenous	N.A.D.	No abnormality demonstrated
KUB	Kidney, Ureter, Bladder		
P.P.	Postpartum	N.P.N.	Non-protein Nitrogen
Pt	Patient	N.Y.D.	Not Yet Diagnosed
P.M.P.	Past Menstrual Period	O.B.	Obstetrics
R.B.C.	Red Blood Cells	O.T.	Occupational Therapy
		P.	Pulse
T.P.R.	Temperature, Pulse, Respiration	P.B.I.	Protein Bound Iodine
T.B.W.	Total Body Water	P.C.V.	Packed Cell Volume
T.U.R.	Transurethral Resection	R.P.F.	Relaxed Pelvic Floor
VD	Veneral Disease		Renal Plasma Flow
VE	Vaginal Examination	S.A.	Sino-atrial
VP	Venous Pressure	S.G.O.T.	Serum Glutamic Oxalacetic Transaminase
XR	X-Ray	S.G.P.T.	Serum Glumatic Pyruvic Transaminase
		S.O.B.	Shortness of Breath
		S.O.L.	Space Occupying Lesion
		S.O.S.	If Necessary
		T.B.	Tuberculosis
		U and C	Urethral and Cervical
		U.R.I.	Upper Respiratory Tract Infection
		U.T.I.	Urinary Tract Infection
		U.S.P.	United States Pharmacopoeia
		W.B.C.	White Blood Cells
		Wt.	Weight
		W.R.	Wassermann Reaction

The Variety of Dosage Forms:

The different forms in which a medicinal agent can be administered for the convenient and efficacious treatment of disease are as follows:

Solid Dosage Forms:

- **Tablets:** The dosage forms of medicinal substances usually prepared with the aid of suitable pharmaceutical adjuncts.
- **Powder:** It is a mixture of finely divided drugs and/or chemicals in dry form.
- **Capsules:** The dosage forms in which one or more medicinal and/or inert substances are enclosed within a small shell or container of gelatine.

- **Pills:** Small, round solid dosage forms containing a medicinal agent and intended to be administered orally.

Liquid Dosage Forms:

- **Solutions:** Liquid preparations containing one or more soluble chemical substances usually dissolved in water.
- **Syrups:** Aqueous saturated solution of sugar.
- **Elixirs:** Sweetened hydroalcoholic solutions.
- **Spirits:** Alcoholic solutions of aromatic materials.
- **Aromatic water:** Aqueous solutions of aromatic materials.
- **Tinctures:** Alcoholic or hydroalcoholic solutions of chemical substances.
- **Suspensions:** Preparations containing finely divided drug particles distributed uniformly throughout a vehicle in which a drug exhibits minimum degree of solubility.
- **Emulsions:** It is a dispersion in which the dispersed phase is composed of small globules of a liquid distribute throughout a vehicle in which it is immiscible.
- **Injections:** These are sterile pyrogen free preparation intended to be administered parenterally.

Semisolid Dosage Forms:

- **Ointments:** These are semisolid dosage forms, greasy in appearance intended for external use only.
- **Lotions:** Lotions are liquid preparations intended for external application to the skin. These dry on the skin soon after application leaving a thin coat of medicament on the skin.
- **Creams:** These are non-greasy semisolid preparations.
- **Poultices:** These are the pastes with a base of kaolin and glycerin for external application in warm conditions.
- **Suppositories:** These are solid dosage forms intended for insertion into body orifices where they melt, soften or dissolve and exert localised or systemic effect.
- **Liniments** These are alcoholic or oleogenous solutions or emulsions of various medicinal substances intented for external application to the skin generally with rubbing.
- **Aerosols:** These are pressurized dosage forms containing one or more active ingredients which upon actuation emit a fine dispersion of liquid and/or solid materials in a gaseous medium.
- **Inhalers:** These are the drugs or solutions of drugs administered by the nasal or oral respiratory route.
- **Sprays:** These are aqueous or oleogenous solutions in the form of coarse droplets or as finely divided solids to be applied topically.

PHARMACEUTICAL LATIN TERMS

Latin Term	Abbreviation	Meaning
1. Dosage forms:		
Tabella or Tabletta	tab.	A Tablet
Capsula	caps.	A Capsule

Latin Term	Abbreviation	Meaning
Pulvis	pulv.	A Powder
Pilula	pil	A pill
Mistura	m, mist.	A mixture
Emulsio	emul.	An emulsion
Liquor	liq.	A solution
Cataplasmatis	cataplasm	A Poultice
Tincture	tinct.	A tincture
Injectio	inj.	An injection
Lotio	lot.	A lotion
Linimentum	lin.	A liniment
Pasta	past.	A paste
Pigmentum	pigm.	A paint
Unguentum	ung.	An ointment
Vapor	vap.	An inhalation
Suspensio	susp.	A suspension
Suppositorium	suppos.	A suppository
Nebula	neb.	A spray solution
Guttae	gtt.	Drops
Gelatina	gelat.	A jelly
Gargarisma	garg.	A gargle
Naristillae	narist	Nasal drops
Auristillae	auristill.	Ear drops
Sternutamentum	Sternut.	A snuff
Collunarium	Collun.	A nose wash
Collutorium	Collut.	A mouth wash
Collyrium	collyr.	An eye lotion
2. Time of administration		
Semel in die	sem. in die	Once a day
Bis in die	b.i.d.	Twice a day
Ter in die	t.i.d.	Thrice a day
Quater in die	q.i.d.	Four times a day
Bis terve in die	b.t.i.d..	Two or three times a day
Ter quaterve die	t.q.d.	Three or four times a day
Quotidie	quot.	Daily
Ter quotidie	ter. quot.	Three times daily
Mane	m.	In the morning
Omni Mane	o.m.	Every morning
Primo mane	prim. m.	Early in the morning
Jentaculum	jentac.	Breakfast
Nocte	n.	At night
Hora somni	h.s.	At bed time
Vespere	vesp.	In the evening

Latin Term	Abbreviation	Meaning
Omni nocte	o.n.	Every night
Cras	–	Tomorrow
Hebdomada	hebdom.	A week
Hora, horis	h.	hour
cibos, cibum	c.	Meal

Abbreviations commonly used in Measure of Capacity and Weight

Symbol	Latin	English	Equal to
Capacity:			
m	Minimum	Minim	1 minim
ʒ or 'f ʒ	Fluidrachma	fl. drachm	60 minim
℥ or 'f ℥	Fluidunicia	fl. flounce	480 minim or 8 fl. drachm
'O'	octarius	pint	16 fl. ounce
'qt'	–	quart	32 fl. ounce
'C'	Congius	gallon	160 fl. ounce
Weight:			
gr	Granum	grain	1 grain
℈	Scrupulus	scruple	20 grain
ʒ	Drachma	drachm	60 grain or 3 scruple
℥	Uncia	ounce	480 grain or 8 drachm
*l*b	Libra	pound	5760 grain or 12 drachm

QUESTIONS

1. Define the terms Medicine, Disease.
2. Give the different types of diseases with examples and their causes.
3. Define the terms: (a) Antimicrobial (b) Antifungal (c) Anti-parasitic (d) Antibiotic.
4. Give the meaning of following abbreviations.
   B.B.T., C.T., D.L.C., E.C.F., E.S.R., D.O.A., F.B.S., I.B.I., K.U.B., L.M.P., M.C.V., N.A.D., S.G.P.T., S.G.O.T., W.N.L. and U.R.T.
5. What are the different dosage forms in which a drug may be placed for treatment of disease?
6. Give the meaning of following latin terms:
   (i) Mistura (vi) Auristillae
   (ii) Lotio (vii) Sternutamentum
   (iii) Unguentum (viii) Vapor
   (iv) Nebula (ix) Gelatina
   (v) Guttae (x) Collutorium.
7. What do you know about following latin abbreviations:
   (i) b.i.d. (ii) t.i.d. (iii) t.q.d. (iv) quot
   (v) o.m. (vi) o.n. (vii) h.s. (viii) prim. m.
8. Give the symbols for the following:
   (i) Drachma (ii) Gallon (iii) Pint (iv) Ounce.

***

4

PATHOPHYSIOLOGY OF DISEASES

It is necessary to understand the pharmacological effects of drugs and the way in which those effects interact with the processes underlying the pathology of the disease. Unfortunately, it is not always possible but we can still try to understand the underlying processes of the disease, that is its "pathophysiology" and base our questions about the role of specific drugs on our understanding of the pathophysiology of the disease and relevant pharmacological effects of the drugs used in its treatment.

The pathophysiological processes involved are illustrated in Fig. 4.1.

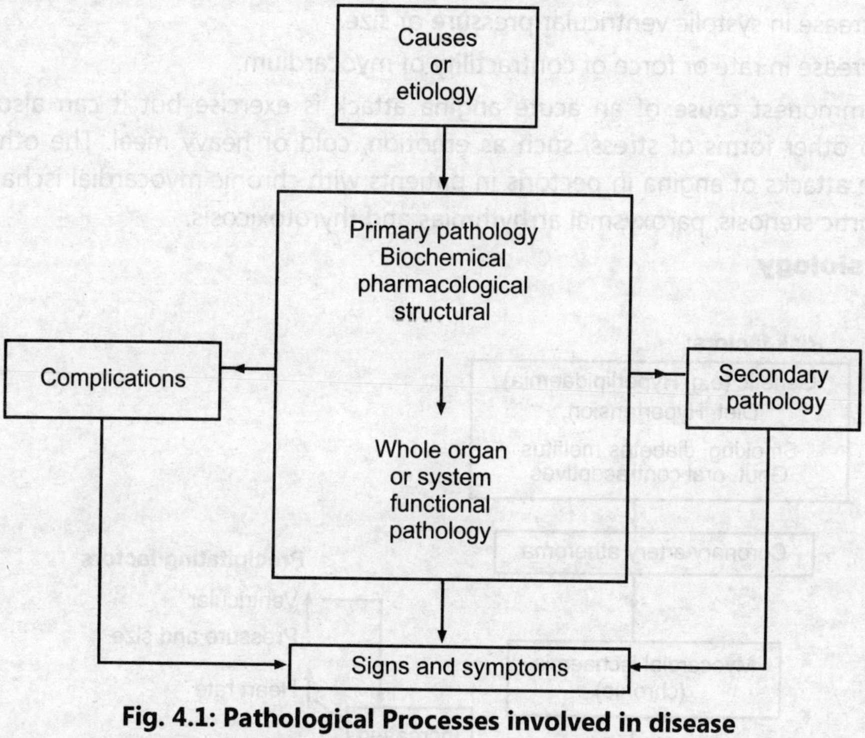

Fig. 4.1: Pathological Processes involved in disease

Consider Pneumococcal pneumonia.

The 'cause' is infection with the pneumococcus.

(Streptococcus pneumoniae)

The *primary pathology* is the inflammatory response resulting in abnormalities in lung function e.g. Hypoxia.

The pleurisy and pleural effusion is the *secondary pathology* and metastatic pneumococcal infection. (e.g. Cerebral abscess) is regarded as complication.

Each of these primary pathology, secondary pathology and complications produces its own signs and symptoms. The symptoms are subjective feelings e.g. Nausea, pain, whereas the objectively identifiable changes are termed as signs e.g. fever, *reddening of the skin*. The detectable structural change produced in the course of disease is known as lesion.

CARDIOVASCULAR DISEASES

(1) Angina Pectoris

The syndrome of angina pectoris occurs when there is an acute imbalance between the oxygen requirements of the myocardium and the oxygen available to it. This occurs either when there is sudden spasm of coronary artery or sudden increase in demand for oxygen in a chronically ischaemic heart. The increase in oxygen demand may result from any stimulus which causes.

(i) Increase in heart rate.

(ii) Increase in systolic ventricular pressure or size.

(iii) Increase in rate or force of contractility of myocardium.

The commonest cause of an acute angina attack is exercise but it can also occur in response to other forms of stress, such as emotion, cold or heavy meal. The other factors which cause attacks of angina in pectoris in patients with chronic myocardial ischaemia are : anaemia, aortic stenosis, paroxysmal arrhythmias and thyrotoxicosis.

Pathophysiology

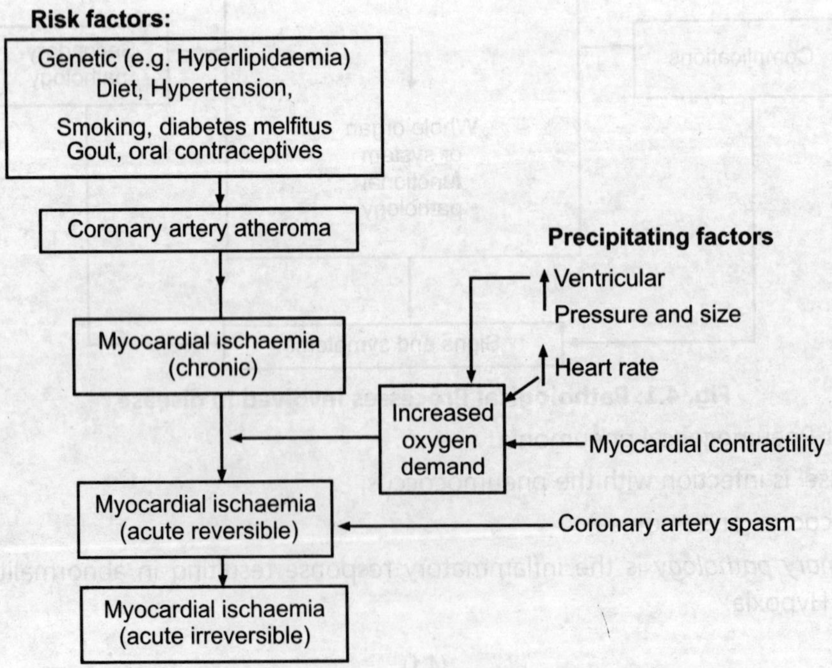

Signs and Symptoms

Pain occurs below the sternum on left side and it radiates to the neck, lower jaw, shoulder and passes down through the left arm. The duration of attack of anginal pain can be from 30 sec. to 45 min.

(2) Congestive Heart Failure

It is caused by the inability of the heart to meet increased demands, namely, the inability of the stroke volume to maintain equality with the volume of blood returned to the heart. As the cardiac muscle loses its ability to keep pace with demand, the pulse rate increases. When the cardiac reserve is exhausted, the pathologic changes result in congestive cardiac failure (C.C.R).

Pathophysiology

The basic pathologic process is increased vascular permeability. The lungs are the seat of pathologic changes when the left side of the heart fails. Increased intravascular pressure is transmitted to the pulmonary capillaries. As these vessels dilate, plasma leaks into surrounding tissues. As time goes on, the leakage of fluid becomes so great that fluid accumulates in alveoli (Pulmonary edema) and pleural space (pleural effusion). Red blood cells may escape from vessels, so that pulmonary edema is blood-tinged. Generalized congestion and edema cause shortness of breath and coughing. The cough may produce blood-tinged sputum. Alveolar lining cells undergo hypertrophy and help to remove the pulmonary edema fluid and fragmented R.B.Cs.

Causes of Cardiac Failure

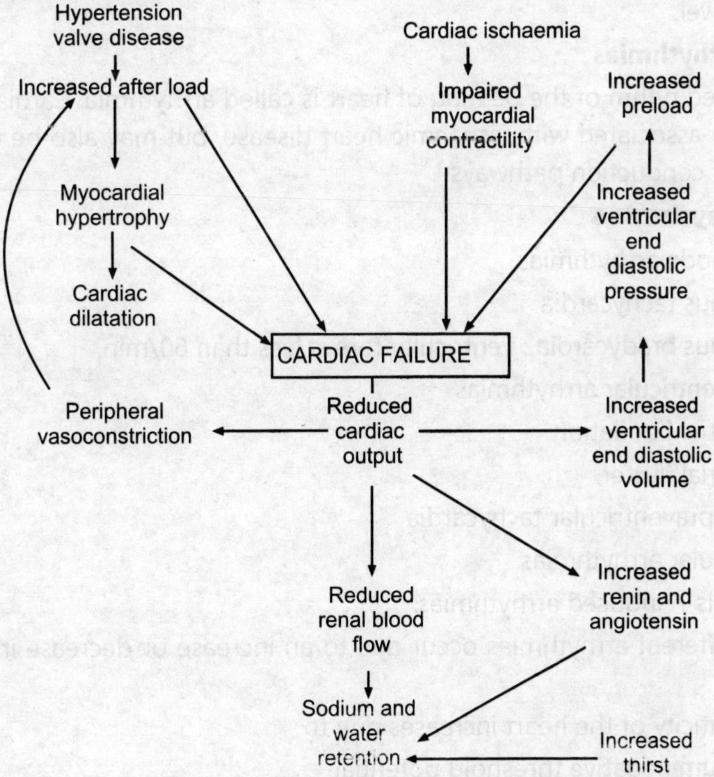

Fig. 4.2: Pathophysiological processes of cardiac failure

1. Decreased contractility due to chronic ischaemia, acute infarction and cardiomyopathies.
2. Increased after load due to hypertension aortic valve disease and hypertrophic obstructive cardiomyopathy.
3. Increased cardiac output due to mitral incompetence, arrhythmias, anemia, hyperthyroidism and peripheral shunts.
4. Pulmonary heart disease due to chronic airway obstruction and pulmonary embolism.

Signs and Symptoms

1. Coughing and shortness of breath.
2. The skin turns bluish i.e. cyanosis.
3. The patient may cough up a frothy, pinkish, blood-tinged material especially at night.
4. Patient becomes anxious and fearful for his own future.
5. Enlargement and tenderness of liver.
6. Kidneys are congested and unable to excrete excess fluid from the body.
7. Presence of albumin and casts in urine.
8. Distressing symptoms such as gas, constipation, lack of appetite and distension of the bowel.

(3) Cardiac Arrhythmias

The disturbed rythm of the beating of heart is called arrhythmia. Cardiac arrhythmias are most commonly associated with ischaemic heart disease, but may also be due to congenital abnormalities of conduction pathways.

Types of Arrhythmias

(a) Sinus node arrhythmias
   (i) sinus tachycardia
   (ii) sinus bradycardia : ventricular rate is less than 60/min.

(b) Supraventricular arrhythmias
   (i) Atrial fibrillation
   (ii) Atrial flutter.
   (iii) Supraventricular tachycardia

(c) Ventricular arrhythmias

(d) Digitallis – induced arrhythmias.

All these different arrhythmias occur due to an increase or decrease in the automaticity of the heart.

The automaticity of the heart increases due to

1. Maximum negative threshold potential,
2. High rate of depolarization,

3. Minimum negative resting potential, and
4. Combination of the above changes.

The automaticity of the heart decreases due to changes opposite to those mentioned above.

(4) Atherosclerosis

It is a morphologic lesion which is yellow to white coloured that appears on the tunica intima of the blood vessel. It is also called as "atheroma". The earliest atheromas are nodular aggregates of smooth muscle cells. The mature atheromas are made up of cellular, fibrous and lipid components. The fatty streaks are perhaps the earliest lesions of atherosclerosis.

Risk Factors in Atherosclerosis

1. Genetic and metabolic factors.
2. **Hypertension:** Both ischaemic heart disease and atherosclerosis are more frequent in hypertensives than in normotensive subjects. Effective treatment of hypertension and cessation of cigarette smoking can reduce atherosclerosis.
3. **Age:** In older subjects incidence of atherosclerosis increases.
4. **Blood lipids:** There is increased incidence of atherosclerosis in patients with increased cholesterol, low density lipoprotein (LDL) and triglycerides with very low density lipoproteins, whereas patients with increased levels of high-density lipoproteins (HDL) are less likely to develop atherosclerosis and ischaemic heart disease.

Manifestations

1. Atherosclerosis of mesenteric vessels may cause abdominal pain and thrombosis in these vessels results in bowel infraction.
2. Pain in legs with loss of hair on legs and weakness of leg muscles.
3. In severe cases it may result in angina pectoris ischaemic renal disease and myocardial infarction.
4. There is extreme sensitivity to cold.

(5) Hypertension

It is the higher than normal increased arterial blood pressure. The hypertension is of two types :

(i) Primary or idiopathic or essential hypertension: The hypertension for which the cause is unknown.

(ii) Secondary hypertension: The cause is known which is due to some definite abnormality.

The severe hypertension may be associated with necrotic vascular changes called as malignant hypertension.

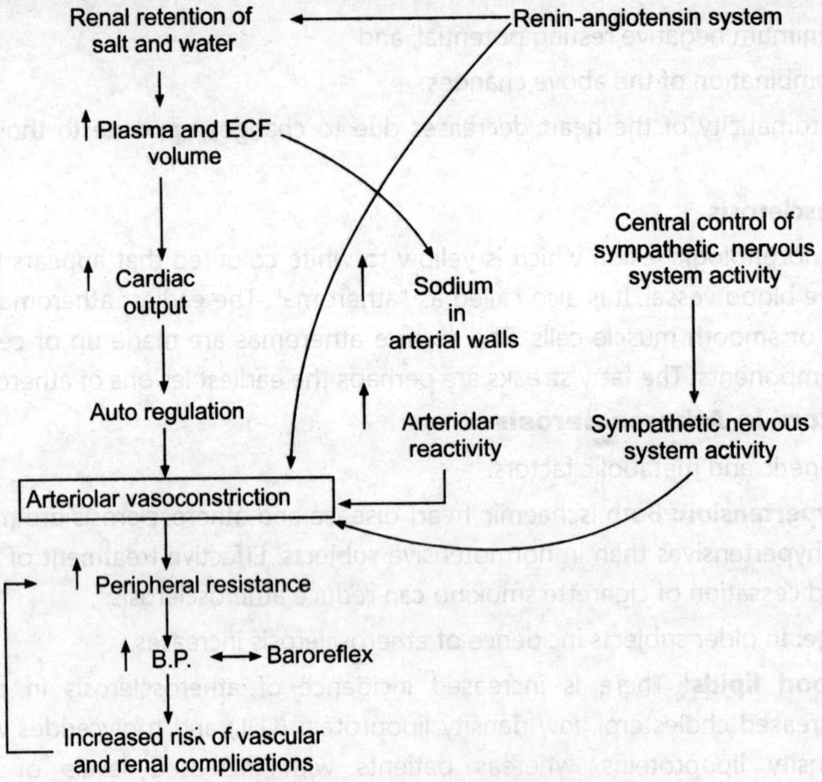

Fig. 4.3: Pathophysiology of hypertension

It is difficult to define precisely degrees of severity of hypertension; a rough working guide is as follows :

(i) Mild hypertension	:	B.P. 130/90 to 140/100 mm of Hg.
(ii) Moderate hypertension	:	B.P. 140/100 to 160/120 mm of Hg.
(iii) Severe hypertension	:	B.P. > 160/120 mm of Hg.
(iv) Hypertensive emergency	:	Diastolic B.P. > 130 mm of Hg.

Pathophysiology

Hypertension affects not only the heart as pathological changes can also occur in eyes, kidneys and brain. Blind spots may interfere with vision because of retinal haemorrhages. Most hypertensive patients have a family background of strokes, heart disease and kidney ailments. The damage to kidney results in retention of salt and water. This increases the volume of plasma and extracellular fluid (E.C.F.), ultimately resulting in increased cardiac output. The increased concentration of sodium in arterial walls increases the arteriolar reactivity causing arteriolar vasoconstriction. The peripheral resistance to blood flow increases causing increase in B.P.

In hypertensive patients there is always a risk of vascular and renal complications leading to increased peripheral resistance.

In renin-angiotensin system of the body, increase in renin secretion causes arteriolar constriction. The sympathetic nervous system activity also causes arteriolar vasoconstriction causing an increase in B.P.

In hypertensive patient, the cardiac output is increased, so the work of the heart is increased causing left ventricular failure. This causes atherosclerosis resulting in hypertension. The brain damage includes cerebral edema, thrombosis and haemorrhage.

Signs and Symptoms

1. Primary aldosteronism which exerts its effect through sodium retention.
2. Cushing's syndrome and phaeochromocytoma.
3. Headaches, the pain especially in back of head and neck.
4. Tiredness and fatigue without any obvious cause.
5. Dizziness especially at the time of sitting up or Eying down.
6. Palpitation of the heart.

(6) Acute Myocardial Infarction (Coronary thrombosis)

Myocardial infarction occurs when there is occlusion of a coronary artery because of thrombosis, spasm or rarely embolism with subsequent irreversible tissue damage.

Pathophysiology

A blood clot may form over part of the inner surface of the heart. Fragments may break off and are carried by the blood stream to the lungs, the brain, kidneys and other organs. The blood clot itself is known as thrombus and broken fragment is called an embolus. If the trouble occurs on the outer wall of the heart, an aneurysm or bulging may occur interfering with the normal action of the heart.

Symptoms :

1. Severe crushing pain in the chest.
2. Feeling of heavy pressure on chest.
3. Pain may continue for hours or days and there may be extreme shortness of breath and possibly nausea, vomitting and hiccups followed by extreme weakness and fear of death.
4. Skin becomes pale, cold and moist and lips bluish in colour.
5. Pulse is weak and slow and may be irregular.

TUBERCULOSIS

Tuberculose (TB) is one of the most serious diseases known to man. Scientist Dr. Koch discovered tubercle bacillus in 1882. The disease is caused by infection with mycobacterium tuberculosis. There are two types of mycobacteria: (1) Human type and (2) Bovine type. Tuberculosis from bovine type is decreased now a days due to pasteurisation of milk and testing of cows.

Pathophysiology

The bacillus that causes tuberculosis is a tiny, rod shaped germ. These germs are protected by an outer layer of wax which prevents the normal defence of the body from destroying them. Tuberculosis may attack any part of the body such as bones, joints, glands, lymph nodes, fallopian tubes, intestine, eyes, kidneys etc. but it specially attacks on lungs causing pulmonary T.B. These germs can live for months in any place especially in a damp area.

These germs are usually spread by coughing and sneezing in the form of water droplets suspended in air.

When the germ enters the lungs, the body defence, i.e. W.B.Cs. surrounds the germs and swallow them. But because of waxy coat, many germs continue to live for months. The larger W.B.Cs. then move in building a wall of resistance against the invaders. This is known as "tubercle".

The tubercle may disappear, leaving a hole or cavity. Large masses of scar tissue may form around these areas. This hinders the flow of blood and interferes with normal functioning of lungs.

Signs and Symptoms

1. Tiredness and fatigue on little or no exertion.
2. Progressive weight loss.
3. Chronic cough and spitting up blood.
4. Chest pain.
5. Night sweats and afternoon fever.
6. Loss of appetite.
7. Weakness and dry mouth.

The diagnosis is made by performing the *tuberculin test*. A small amount of liquid (i.e. tuberculin containing protein fraction of bacillus) is injected into the skin. If it becomes red and inflamed, it indicates the presence of tuberculosis.

HEPATITIS

Hepatitis is an acute inflammation of the liver, caused by viral infection or toxic agent. The term 'viral hepatitis' refers to the primary infection of the liver by hepatitis virus type A or type B or by other hepatitis viruses referred to as 'non-A and non-B'.

Pathophysiology

Type A hepatitis (Infectious hepatitis)

It occurs either sporadically or in epidemics affecting many children and young adults. It is transmitted by fecal-oral route.

The virus enters the body by ingestion and multiplies in the intestinal epithelium before it reaches the liver by haematogenous spread. It is shed in the faeces during the late incubation period and the prodromal phase of the illness. Once jaundice develops, it is rarely detectable in faeces. The virus is present in the blood for a brief period during the pre-icteric stage, but usually disappears, when jaundice sets in. The incubation period is 2 to 6 weeks. The disease consists of two stages viz. prodromal or pre-icteric stage and icteric stage.

Signs and Symptoms

The disease begins with nausea, vomitting, fever, genera weakness and loss of appetite and liver tenderness.

The disease continues for 10 days to 2 weeks and then tends to disappear. There may be enlargement of spleen, itching of skin and diarrhoea.

Type B Hepatitis (Serum hepatitis)

It was originally considered to be an unusual disease transmitted exclusively by *parenteral route* and by iatrogenic procedures such as blood transfusion or injection of serum or other blood products. It is now known to be transmitted also by many natural mechanisms that transfer minute quantities of blood or tissue fluid between persons.

The incubation period is long i.e. 2 to 6 months. Clinically the disease is similar to type A hepatitis but is usually more severe. The onset is insidious and fever is not prominent.

Signs and Symptoms

Rash, arthralgia, polyarteritis nodosa and glomerulonephritis are the symptoms that results from antigen-antibody reaction in the body. Some patients progress to chronic active hepatitis and cirrhosis.

The hepatitis B virus is a DNA virus. Its core of double stranded DNA is enclosed in a lipoprotein coat. The hepatitis virus (HBV) replicates in the liver cells and virus cells or their fragments get incorporated in the liver cell membranes. Several antigenic components are recognised viz.

HB_c Ag (core antigen)

HB_s Ag (surface antigen)

HB_e Ag (also found in the core)

These antigens are responsible for producing the antibodies viz. Ig G and Ig M. These antibodies attack foreign plasma membranes and thus the immune system damages the liver. Persistence of antigen is seen in immunosuppression and in patients with chronic aggressive disease.

DIABETES

Diabetes is of two types: viz. (i) Diabetes mellitus and (ii) Diabetes insipidus.

Diabetes mellitus occurs due to deficiency of insulin whereas diabetes insipidus occurs due to deficiency of ADH (Antidiuretic hormone).

Diabetes mellitus is the condition arising from the abnormal metabolism of carbohydrates, proteins and fats due to deficiency of insulin. Diabetes mellitus clinically is of two types:

(i) Non-insulin dependent or Type-I (Ketoacidosis resistant) diabetes: This is milder form of the disease. There is some defect in the gluco-receptor of the β-cell membrane, which accounts for the delay in secretion of insulin. Disease occurs in adults and obese persons.

(ii) Insulin dependent or Type-II (Ketoacidosis prone) diabetes: It occurs in childhood and the individual is dependent on exogenous insulin to prevent ketoacidosis. Pancreas contains little or no extractable insulin. The main cause is the damage of β-cells in pancreas by invasion of one of the viruses. Persons laving diabetic relatives are more susceptible to such a damage of β-cells. The important symptoms of this diabetes are loss of body weight increased urination, excessive thirst, nausea, bed-wetting, weakness and, itching of skin. The symptoms are relieved by injection of insulin. This is a severe form of the disease.

Pathophysiology

The following equation illustrates how the blood glucose level is maintained within normal limits by the Islets of Langerhans of pancreas.

$$\text{Glucose} \underset{\substack{\text{Glucagon} \\ \text{Glycogenolysis}}}{\overset{\substack{\text{Glycogenesis} \\ \text{Insulin}}}{\rightleftharpoons}} \text{Glycogen}$$

Glucagon also stimulates the process of gluconeogenesis. The various actions of insulin are as follows :

1. It increases the glucose uptake by muscle and fat.
2. It inhibits gluconeogenesis.
3. Conversion of glucose to glycogen and fatty acids promoted.
4. Conversion of fatty acids to triglycerides promoted and reverse reactions inhibited.
5. Conversion of aminoacids to proteins promoted and reverse reactions inhibited.

The normal fasting blood sugar level lies between 80 and 120 mg% whereas after meal it rises to 150 mg%.

Due to low levels of insulin, there is mobilisation of fatty acids leading to formation of ketone bodies and acidosis (keto-acidosis). There is hyperglycaemia and glycosuria resulting in dehydration.

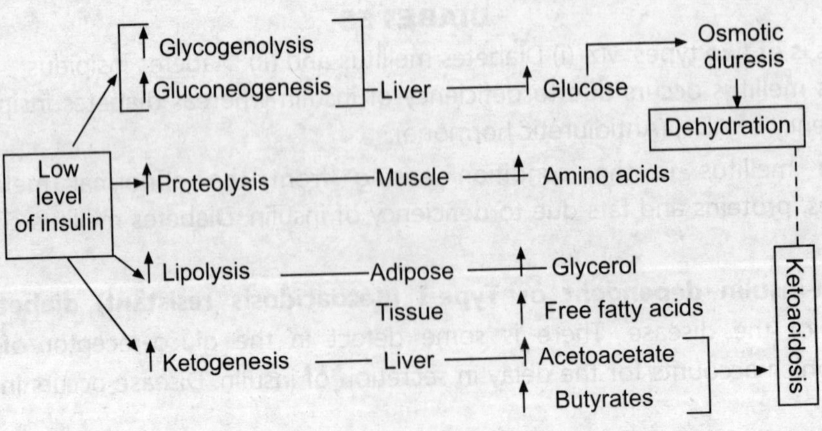

Manifestations (Signs and Symptoms)

Hyperglycemia, glycosuria, polyuria, polydipsia, ketonemia, ketonuria, polyphagia azoturia, poor wound healing and maximum susceptibility to infection and weight loss.

The blood glucose is raised to 600-800 mg%. The blood pH is lowered and the carbon dioxide combining power of blood is markedly reduced. Acute insulin resistance may develop.

Nocturia, blurred vision, neuropathy, nephropathy, vascular complications, numbness in feet are symptoms observed in long term diabetics.

Complications

1. **Ketoacidosis:** The body prefers to use sugar for energy but when it is not available, fat is utilized. When fat is utilized, certain acid substances are produced, known as ketone bodies. These disturb the normal acid-base balance resulting in severe acidosis.
2. **Obesity:** Insulin therapy without dietary restrictions may lead to obesity.
3. **Arteriosclerosis:** Hardening of arteries occurs much more frequently in diabetic patients. This happens particularly in lower extremities where deep *ulcers* may form in the feet or legs and *gangrene* may result from secondary infection.
4. **Cataracts:** Occur more frequently in older diabetics. Diabetic retinitis occurs more frequently in children.
5. **Infections:** Diabetic are more susceptible to infections of skin such as boils, carbuncles and generalized itching.
6. **Nephropathy:** One of the most serious complications is the damage to kidney. Albuminuria, hypertension and oedema of various parts of body occurs.
7. **Hypoglycemia:** The hypoglycemia may result from overdosage of insulin, failure to eat or ingestion of alcohol.
8. Insulin allergy and resistance may develop.

RHEUMATOID ARTHRITIS

Rheumatoid arthritis is a serious disease that involves not only joints but also the muscles, tendons and other tissues of the body. The etiology of the disease is unknown but it occurs more frequently in women.

Pathophysiology

The disease usually begins rather mildly with some swelling, pain and tenderness in the joints of the fingers, knees, wrist and feet. The joints on both sides of the body may be involved simultaneously. The joints may contain some fluid and these feel warm and appear red. During active phase of disease, the patient complains of fatigue, weakness and pain.

Because of the pain, the muscle spasm occurs which create a real problem. The flexor muscles of hand are stronger than the extensor muscles so that the prolonged muscle spasm pulls the joint somewhat out of shape. Other muscles may show atrophic changes. The bones become thinner causing osteoporosis and cartilage may shrivel up.

The patient may become anaemic because of the depression of bone marrow. The course of the disease is quite variable individually. The disease may last for many years and most patients complain of painful joints and muscles.

The drugs which modify the disease process in rheumatoid arthritis are penicillamine, gold salts (sodium aurothiomalate), chloroquine, corticosteroids and immunosuppressive drugs (azathioprine).

Penicillamine affects the production of some immunoglobulins, decreases the concentration of circulating immune complexes (complex formed by antigen-antibody reaction), suppresses lymphocyte stimulation by some agents and improves neutrophil chemotaxis.

The gold salts reduce the circulating concentration of rheumatoid factor and immunoglobulins.

The immune complexes formed in the body react with the complement (the complement system is an interacting system of 18 plasma proteins) cascade resulting in the inflammatory response.

Manifestations

1. Anemia due to suppression of bone marrow.
2. Weight loss, anorexia, muscle fatigue.
3. Stiffness of joints especially in the morning.
4. Deformity of the joint, altered shape of bones, especially of the fingers.
5. Formation of rheumatic nodules on the joints.
6. Inflammation of other vital organs of the body like heart, lungs and eyes also occurs.

PEPTIC ULCER

Ulceration is the loss of the epithelial surface that lines the digestive organs with extension of necrosis into underlying tissues. Peptic ulcer occur in sites where acid pepsin secretion is abundant. The two generally occurring forms of peptic ulcer are: (i) Gastric ulcer and (ii) Duodenal ulcer.

Pathophysiology

The two main factors involved in the pathogenesis of peptic ulceration are:

(i) Acid and pepsin secretion.

(ii) Mucosal resistance to acid and pepsin.

(1) Gastric Ulcer

1. The acid secretion is less than that of patients with duodenal ulcer.
2. Mucous membrane in the stomach of patients with gastric ulcer have less resistance than to those of other subjects.
3. Materials refluxing from the duodenum damage the gastric mucosa.
4. There is increased bile acid in the stomach of patients with gastric ulcer as compared to normal individuals. But there is no direct evidence to support the idea that bile acids damage gastric mucous membranes. Ulceration takes place in any part of stomach.

(2) Duodenal Ulcer

Secretion is stimulated by gastrin and cholinergic postganglionic vagal fibres. Patients have higher acid secretion than normal individuals or patients with gastric ulcer. This increased acid secretion may be due to increase in parietal cell mass or mass of cells responsive to secretory stimuli.

For unknown reasons the incidence of duodenal ulcers are higher in cigarette smokers and in patients with chronic renal failure and alcoholic cirrhosis.

The ulceration usually takes place on the anterior wall of the first portion of duodenum.

Manifestations

Peptic ulcers are usually less than 4 cm in diameter and are round lesions. Its walls are sharply perpendicular and its base is smooth. The ulcer may perforate the wall, extending into adjacent structures. There is fibrosis and scarring with progression of the lesion. Vessels can be seen at the base of ulcer which cause massive bleeding, i.e. haemorrhage and shock.

The most common symptom of ulcer is sharp and severe pain. The patient can always put his finger on the sore spot. In case of duodenal ulcer the pain occurs when the patient is hungry and it may be severe enough to awaken him at night. The pain is relieved by taking alcohol or coffee whereas in case of gastric ulcer pain is relieved by taking food. Due to this a patient gains weight. Diet is most important in the treatment of ulcers. During acute stage, liquid diet such as milk should be given which provides proteins and calcium in adequate quantities to support healing process. Patients not responding to good medical treatment are often advised to have surgery.

Some patients of ulcer may show the presence of blood in vomit and tarry stools. Peritonitis may also occur if ulcer has eroded, allowing the gastric juice to spill out into the abdomen.

EPILEPSY

Epilepsy is a serious disorder characterised by abnormal electrical changes occuring in brain that result in periods of unconsciousness. These periods last from few seconds to several minutes.

Types of Epilepsies

1. Partial seizure: The paroxysmal discharge spreads, locally from a focus of abnormal cells.
2. Grand mal seizures (generalised convulsion).
3. Petit mal seizures (typical absence).

1. Partial Seizure (focal seizure): These are the minor psychomotor attacks in which the patient loses contact with his environment for about 1 to 2 min. He does not fall but may perform automatic purposeless movements. During the attack he does not understand what is said and may oppose any aid. The manifestations of partial seizures depend on the site of origin of discharge. The initial manifestation will be contraction of muscles on opposite side of the body. (Since decussation of nerves in medulla oblongata). The threshold of excitation of cells in motor cortex is lowest for cells which supply the index finger and thumb the corner of mouth or the big toe. Not only the threshold of excitation of these cells is lowest but also there are more cells assigned to control these muscles which are concerned with facial expression. Hence abnormal events occur in these cells.

Manifestations

The first sign of such a seizure is twitching at one corner of mouth. As the discharge spreads the muscles around the eyes, then muscles of hand and then of foot get involved. This type of seizure is often called as Jacksonian Seizure. The person may be confused and mentally clouded for a minute or two after the attack is over.

2. **Grand mal seizures:** Loss of consciousness takes place. The cerebral neurons are connected to other neurons in the spinal cord. The axons of some of these pass through nerves to innervate muscles. The powerful generalized cortical seizure discharge is therefore linked through this direct transmission system to muscle fibres. Discorded contraction of all muscles is the cause of a grand mal seizure.

Manifestations

(i) **Tonic phase:** The first phase of grand malseizure is known as *tonic (contraction) phase*. Due to widespread contraction of muscles, the body is rigid and incapable of maintaining a normal posture, so that subject falls to the ground.

(ii) **Crying:** The respiratory muscles also contract, forcing out the air through the larynx. So there may be involuntary noise i.e. a grunt or a cry at the onset of the attack.

(iii) **Bleeding in mouth:** The jaw muscles also contract and during severe muscular spasms, the normal muscular movements that keep the tongue out of the way are disordered and the tongue or cheek may be bitten leading to bleeding.

(iv) **Cyanosis** of face due to strong contraction of the chest muscles.

(v) **Frothing at mouth:** Normal movements of swallowing are lost so that saliva dribbles out between the tightly clenched teeth.

(vi) **Mydriasis and seating may occur.**

(vii) **Incontinence of urine:** The disordered contraction of abdominal and bladder muscles may result in incontinence of urine.

The second phase viz. clonic or convulsive phase follows after one or two minutes of tonic phase with rythmic movements of limbs and trunk muscles. These gradually cease after a few minutes and subject lies passively unconscious. Normal colour returns, consciousness lightens and the subject can be roused. After this, he will be confused and restless. He may suffer a headache for the rest of the day or may sleep for a couple of hours.

- Dilantin sodium, 100 mg once or twice a day or Phenobarbital $\frac{1}{4}$ to $\frac{1}{2}$ grain 2-3 times a day is sufficient to keep patient free from attacks.

3. Petit Mal Seizures (Typical absence): These are associated with characteristic electro-encaphalographic discharges. It is a disorder of childhood. A typical attack is very brief, lasting only a few seconds. It is less serious form of epilepsy and the loss of consciousness is momentary. The child may suddenly stop, what he is doing, stare, flutter his eyelids and drop his head slightly forward. The posture of the limbs and trunk is usually maintained so that child does not fall. These attacks may be unobserved by the parents and the child resumes what he has been doing after the attack. It is often associated with myoclonic jerks. The petit mal seizures may be very frequent i.e. 10-50 seizures a day.

- Tridione many times a day is useful for this seizure.

Status epilepticus is a phrase used to indicate seizures occurring so close together that one seizure runs into another, without recovery of normal cerebral function between seizures. It may happen with any type of seizure and called as petit mal status, temporal lobe status, or grand mal status. The grand mal status epilepticus is a medical emergency in which the subject does not recover consciousness.

QUESTIONS

1. What are the pathological processes involved in disease ?
2. Give the causes of cardiac failure.
3. Name the risk factors and precipitating factors for 'Angina Pectoris'.
4. Describe the pathophysiological process of angina pectoris and C.C.F.
5. Give the signs and symptoms of cardiac failure.
6. Name the different types of cardiac arrhythmias.
7. What is atherosclerosis ? Give its risk factors.
8. What is hypertension ? Give its types and symptoms.
9. Describe the pathophysiological processes of hypertension.
10. What do you mean by mild, moderate and severe hypertension ?
11. Explain the pathophysiology and manifestations of coronary thrombosis.
12. Describe the pathophysiology and manifestations of tuberculosis. What is the significance of tuberculin test ?
13. What is hepatitis ? Give its types and symptoms.
14. Name the causative organisms for the following with their incubation period :
    (i) Tuberculosis, (ii) Hepatitis.

15. What is diabetes mellitus ? Give its types. What is the normal blood glucose level ?
16. What are the various actions of insulin ?
17. Describe the pathophysiology and symptoms of diabetes mellitus.
18. Give the complications in the treatment of diabetes mellitus.
19. What is rheumatoid arthritis ? Describe its pathophysiology and manifestations.
20. Define peptic ulcer. Classify it.
21. Describe the pathophysiology of peptic ulcer ?
22. What are the signs and symptoms of peptic ulcer ?
23. What is epilepsy ? What are its different types ? Describe its pathophysiology.
24. Give the signs and symptoms of grand mal seizures.
25. What is status epilepticus ?

***

5

PHYSIOLOGICAL PARAMETERS

There are certain physiological constants of the human body which are determined for the evaluation of health status and for diagnosis of disease.

I. Pulse Rate or Heart Rate

Pulse is defined as the wave of expansion and elongation produced in the wall of aorta and passed on to all the arteries of the body. The pulse may be palpated by pressing the artery against the underlying bone. Thus it can be observed on the radial, brachial, axillary, femoral, carotid and temporal arteries. Usually the radial artery at wrist is used.

The normal pulse rate in adults is – 60 to 80/min.

Neonates	–	130-140/min
Children	–	100-130/min
Adults	–	65 to 80 /min.

Significance: It helps in assessing the myocardial status and character of B.P. It increases in the following conditions: Emotional excitement, fever, exercise, metabolic rate, respiration and size of animal. Increase in heart rate is called as tachycardia and decrease is called as bradycardia.

II. Body temperature

The "Clinical Thermometer" is used for measurement of body temperature. The bulb of clinical thermometer is kept at various body positions for specific time. The temperature recorded at the end of 1 min. is body temperature. The normal body temperature is 37.5°C.

Significance: Increase in body temperature is the most common symptom of illness. Thus, it indicates the status of health.

III. Clotting Time of Blood

It is the time taken for the development of fibrin thread from the time blood escapes from the vessels.

Normal clotting time of blood is 3 to 6 min.

Significance: It is important to detect the clotting time of blood before doing any major surgery. According to the necessity, drugs can be administered to prevent excessive loss of blood. It is used in the diagnosis of disease like haemophilia (delay in clotting), haemorrhage, jaundice, leukemia, anemia. Decreased clotting time may result in intravascular clotting of blood called as thrombosis and embolism.

IV. Blood Pressure

The instrument used for measurement of blood pressure is called as sphygmomanometer.

Sphygmomanometers are of two types:

(i) Mercury manometer,

(ii) Aneroid type manometer.

The normal blood pressure is described as 120/80 mm of Hg. Systolic B.P. ranges from 100-150 mm of Hg.

Diastolic B.P. ranges from 60-90 mm of Hg.

The difference between systolic and diastolic pressures is known as pulse pressure which ranges from 45 to 50 mm of Hg.

The increase in systolic B.P. above 150 mm of Hg and diastolic B.P. above 95 mm of Hg is called hypertension and decrease in the above values is called as hypotension.

As the age advances the B.P. increases. The value of B.P. in mm of Hg are:

Infants	–	60/40
Children	–	100/70
Adults	–	120/80

After age of 20 years systolic B.P. may rise 0.5 mm of Hg for each year of age.

Significance: Blood pressure determination is a good aid in the diagnosis of disease. Diastolic B.P. represents the mean B.P. and a state of peripheral resistance which ultimately determines the strain on the vascular system. Systolic B.P. is decreased in conditions like shock, peripheral vasodilation and anaemias. The cardiac output and elasticity of blood vessels are useful for maintaining the systolic B.P. But in conditions like atherosclerosis, diabetes mellitus and in aged peoples, the systolic B.P. increases without change in cardiac output.

Some Diseases Related to B.P.

Systolic B.P.	Diastolic B.P.	Disease
1. 90-100 mm of Hg	150-160 mm of Hg	Hypertension
2. Normal	Higher	Emotion, Atherosclerosis, thyrotoxicosis.
3. Lower	Higher	Aortic regurgitation, patient ductus arteriosus.
4. Lower	Lower	Aortic stenosis, myocardial infarction, pulmonary tuberculosis, anaemia.
5. Higher	Higher	Nephritis, Unilateral kidney disease: Cystic, Hydro, Pyleo, Stone.

B.P. may rise due to:

(i) High sodium/fat intake in the diet.

(ii) Glomerulonephritis.

(iii) Cushing's syndrome.

(iv) Pheochromocytoma.

V. Haemoglobin Count

Normal range:

Male : 15.5 ± 2.5 gm %

Female : 14.0 ± 2.5gm %

Infant : 16.5 ± 3.0 gm %

Significance: The count of haemoglobin decreases in anaemia and leukemia, while increases in dehydration and polycythemia.

V. R.B.C. Count

Normal range:

Male : 4.5 to 5.5 millions per cu. mm

Female : 3.5 to 5.5 millions per cu. mm

Infant : 4.0 to 5.5 millions per cu. mm

Significance: R.B.C. count increases in the following conditions - High altitudes, fasting, sweating, vomitting, diarrhoea, polyuria, defective oxygenation in lungs, severe burns, congenital heart diseases.

The count decreases in all types of anaemias and leukemias and after haemorrhage.

VII. W.B.C. Count (Total Leucocyte Count)

Normal count:

Adults : 6,000 to 10,000 per cu. mm

Children : 8,000 to 10,000 per cu. mm

Infants : 10,000 to 20,000 per cu. mm

Clinical significance:

Leucopenia : Count below 4,000 per cu. mm

Leucocytosis : Count increases to 11,000- 20,000 per cu. mm

Leukaemia (Blood cancer) : Count beyond 20,000 - 1,00,000 per cu. mm

Leucocytosis: Occurs in the following conditions:

1. Asthma, hay fever and skin diseases.
2. Appendicitis, tonsilitis, meningitis, convulsions.
3. Diabetic coma, uraemia, gout lead-poisoning.
4. **Physiological:** Muscular exercise, fear, increased adrenal cortex activity, pregnancy, menstruation, after a meal.
5. Acute infection by pyogenic cocci.

Leucopenia: Occurs in the following conditions:

1. Starvation, fear, anxiety or stress.
2. Blood disorders like agranulocytosis, aplastic anemia and lymphatic leukemias.
3. Influenza, measles and enteric fever.
4. Exposure to UV radiations.
5. Hepatitis, cirrhosis.

VIII. Differential Leucocyte Count (DLC)

The proportion of different types of leucocytes is as follows:

Neutrophils (Polymorphs)	-	60-70%
Eosinophils	-	2-4%
Basophils	-	0-2%
Lymphocytes	-	20-30%
Monocytes	-	5-10%

Significance:

Neutrophillia: (Increase of neutrophils)

1. Acute bacterial infections like pneumonia, whooping cough, septicemia, appendicitis.
2. Neutrophils appear in urine of patients with urinary tract infection.
3. Intoxication or some infections show increase in number of nuclear lobes.

Eosinophillia (Increase of eosinophils):

It indicates the allergic condition and presence of intestinal parasites. In asthma of the bronchial type, renal or cardiac, the count increases. It is also observed in many skin diseases. Eosinopenia (Decrease of eosinophils) occurs in injuries, burns or release of adrenocortical hormones and in acute pyogenic infections.

Basophillia - occurs in granulocytic leukemia.

Lymphocytosis (Increase of lymphocytes)

Acute infections like measles, mumps, influenza. Patients with chronic lymphatic leukemia, tuberculosis and whooping cough show extremely high counts. Conditions like enteric fever and diabetes also show higher count.

Monocytosis (Increase of monocytes)

1. Bacterial infections: Tuberculosis, bacterial endocarditis.
2. Protozoal infections: Malaria.
3. Monocytic leukemia.
4. Hodgkin's disease.

IX. Erythrocyte Sedimentation Rate (E.S.R.)

ESR is defined as millimetre of clear plasma formed at the top of the vertical column in one hour.

Normal value: It is measured in mm/hour.

Method	E.S.R. mm/hour	
	Male	Female
Westergren	3-5	4-7
Wintrobe	0-9	2-20

Significance: The E.S.R. determination is of great importance in the diagnosis of diseases like tuberculosis and rheumatoid arthritis in which it increases. The E.S.R. also increases in anemia, jaundice and septicemia. The E.S.R. decreases in allergic condition.

X. Blood Sugar

Normal value: Fasting blood sugar is 80-120 mg/100 ml. Increase in blood sugar is known as hyperglycemia and decrease in blood sugar is known as hypoglycemia.

Significance: Blood sugar level rarely exceeds 200 mg % except in diabetes.

Hypoglycemia may be the result of insulin overdose, pancreatic tumor or alcohol intake.

XI. Blood Cholesterol

Normal value: 115 to 250 mg %

As age increases, the blood cholesterol increases and it may rise upto 300 mg %.

Cholesterol in the blood is present as

(i) Free cholesterol - 30% of total cholesterol (20-40%) and

(ii) Ester cholesterol - 70% of total cholesterol (60-80%)

Significance

Total Cholesterol level mg %	Disease
300-400	Coronary thrombosis
400-500	Diabetes
500-700	Obstructive jaundice
600-700	Nephrosis
80-100	Hyperthyroidism, pernicious anemia

Percentage of ester cholesterol decreases in diabetes, nephrosis, jaundice and myxedema.

XII. Sperm Count

Normal value: 50 to 150 millions per c.c.

Significance: Useful for detecting the productivity. Persons with less sperm count may show infertility.

XIII. Urine Analysis

A. Physical Tests	Male	Female
1. Colour	Faint yellow	All these indicates the urine sample is physiological. Otherwise the sample is pathological.
2. Appearance	Clear	
3. Odour	Aromatic	
4. Volume	350-500 ml	
5. Specific gravity	1.02-1.03	
6. Reaction	Slightly acidic	
B. Chemical Tests	**Normal Value**	**Significance**
1. Protein (Albumin)	Abnormal constituent	Proteinuria (Albuminuria) Nephritis Pyelonephritis Pregnancy High protein meal
2. Sugar (Glucose)	Abnormal constituent	Glycosuria (Diabetes)
3. **Bile Salts:** Sodium taurocholate Sodium glycocholate **Bile pigments:** Billirubin Billiverdin	Abnormal constituent	Jaundice
4. Ketone bodies	Abnormal constituent	Ketonuria (ketosis) Hypoglycemia
5. Blood cells	Abnormal constituent	Haematuria Acute inflammation of urinary organs, cancer, kidney stone, haemolysis due to poisons.
C. Microscopic Tests	**Normal Value**	**Significance**
1. R.B.Cs	–	Damage to glomerular filters. Tumor of bladder/ kidney Nephritis Bleeding lesion in the urinary tract.
2. Pus cells	–	R.B.C. with pus indicates pyelonephritis
3. Crystals	Appears after long time	–
4. Epithelial cells	Traces in normal urine	Haemorrhagic and degenerative nephritis.
5. Casts	Traces in normal urine	Renal irritation causes increased amounts.

XIV. C.S.F. Examination

Test	Normal Value	Significance
Properties:	It is a clear, colourless fluid which does not clot on standing. The specific gravity is 1.003 and the cells present are only lymphocytes with count of 6 per cu.mm.	
1. Colour	**Abnormal:** Brownish	Presence of blood due to subarachnoid haemorrhage.
	Yellow	Due to haemoglobin conversion to billirubin or because of spinal tumor or increased protein level in C.S.F.
2. Turbidity	Abnormal	Presence of great number of cells, or organisms cause turbidity e.g. Pneumococcal meningitis. Presence of few R.B.Cs. cause smoky appearance to C.S.F.
3. Coagulum	Abnormal	1. If C.S.F. is allowed to stand overnight, it forms 'clot' indicating the disease TB. 2. C.S.F. solidifies on standing in patients with spinal tumor. 3. Great increase of proteins in C.S.F. gives fibrin clots on standing.
4. Microscopic Test Cells:	Only few 0-5 W.B.Cs/cu.mm	If R.B.Cs. are present, observe whether crenated or normocytic.
5. Chemical Test: (a) Protein	15-45 mg %	Increased protein content manifests the inflammation, toxicity, tumors of brain and spinal chord.
(b) Glucose	40-70 mg % in fasting adult	If C.S.F. sugar decreases then it indicates meningitis. 10-25 mg % suppurative meningitis. 20-40 mg % Tuberculous meningitis. 30-45 mg % syphilis meningitis. C.S.F. glucose level increases to 70-100 mg% in diabetes mellitus, brain tumors and encephalitis.
(c) Chlorides	650-750 mg %	The C.S.F. chlorides decrease to 600 mg % or sometimes to 450 mg % in tuberculous meningitis. Hence, useful in diagnosis.

XV. Stool Examination

Tests	Normal Value	Significance
A. Physical Test:		
1. Consistency	Semisolid	Liquid stools in pathogenic bacterial and amoeba infections.
2. Colour	Brownish due to stercobilin	Internal haemorrhage may change the colour.
3. Odour	Characteristics due to indole and skatole	Ulceration in rectum may give foul odour.
4. Mucous	Very less amount	Excessive loss in conditions like dysentry, amoebiasis and colitis.
B. Microscopic Test:		
1. Cells	–	Amoebic dysentry R.B.Cs, mucous and pus cells. Bacillary dysentry Macrophages and Pus cells.
2. Crystals	–	Ulcerative lesions of intestine shows colourless Ca-oxalate, Ca-carbonate crystals of needle shaped. Haemorrhage: Brownish needs.
3. Parasites and eggs	–	Various protozoal like *E. coli* and worms are present in the stool.
C. Chemical Examination: Similar to Urine Analysis		

Some Other Physiological Values

1. Bleeding time (Duke's method) - 0 to 7 min
2. Blood volume - 65-85 ml/kg
3. Packed cell volume (haematorcrit value)
   - Men - 40-55%
   - Women - 35-50%
4. pH of blood - 7.35-7.45
5. Prothrombin time - 10 to 14 seconds

Chemical substance	Quantity in plasma/serum
1. Alkali reserve	55 - 70 ml % CO_2
2. Bilirubin	0.1 - 0.8 mg %
3. Calcium	9 - 11 mg %
4. Chloride	340 - 400 mg %
	140 - 280 mg %
5. Iron	0.08 - 0.20 mg %
6. Magnesium	1.5 - 3 mg %
7. Nitrogen, non-protein	20 - 30 mg %
total	1.05 - 1.4 mg %
8. Potassium	14.8 - 20.2 mg %
	(3.8 - 5.2 m Eq/lit.)
9. Protein total	6 to8.5 g %
albumin	3.5 - 6 g %
globulin	1.5 - 3 g %
fibrinogen	200 - 400 mg %
10. Serum glutamic oxaloacetic transaminase (SGOT)	8 to 40 Spectrophotometric units/ml
11. Serum glutamic pyruvic transaminase (SGPT)	5-35 spectrophotometric units/ml
12. Urea	18 - 40 mg %
13. Uric acid	1.5 - 6.6 mg %
14. Sodium	301 - 340 mg %
	(135 - 138 M Eq/lit.)
15. Phosphatase, acid	0 - 3 King Armstrong units per 100 ml
16. Phosphatase, alkali	3 - 13 King Armstrong units per 100 ml

QUESTIONS

1. Give the normal physiological values for the following:
   (a) Blood cholesterol
   (b) Blood pressure
   (c) E.S.R.
   (d) Haemoglobin
   (e) R.B.C.
   (f) W.B.C.
   (g) Blood sodium
   (h) Blood potassium
   (i) S.G.P.T.
   (j) S.G.O.T.

2. Give the clinical significance of
   (a) Blood pressure
   (b) E.S.R.
   (c) D.L.C.
   (d) Clotting time
   (e) Blood cholesterol
3. Name the abnormal constituents of urine with their clinical significance.
4. Describe the microscopic examination of stool and its significance.
5. What is normal blood glucose level? What is its clinical significance?
6. What is the normal CSF glucose level? Give its clinical significance.
7. What is the significance of CSF chlorides?
8. Describe the physical examination of urine and stool.

***

6

DRUG INTERACTIONS

Drug interactions can occur inside or outside the body; called as *in-vivo* and *in-vitro* drug interactions. The term *in-vitro* drug interaction is referred to as incompatibilities. *In-vitro* drug interactions occur, when two or more drugs are administered simultaneously and these also include:

(a) Drug-food interactions.

(b) Drug-disease interactions.

(c) Drug-environmental chemical (e.g. *smoking)* interactions.

(d) Drug-laboratory test interaction.

Various Sites of Drug Interactions

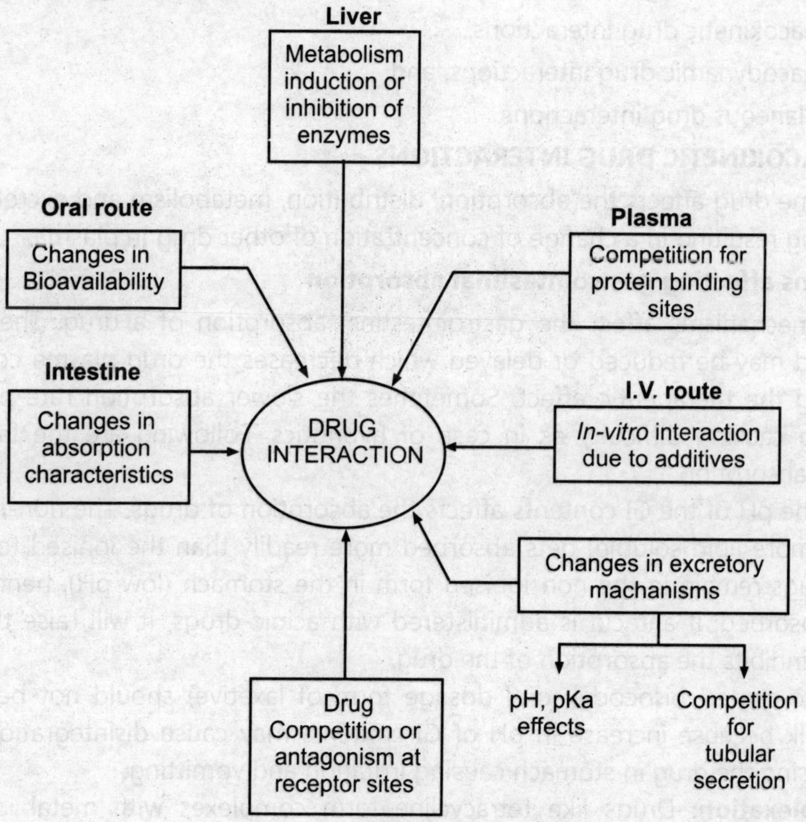

Fig. 6.1

Causes of Drug Interactions

Various factors are responsible for the drug interactions.

1. **Use of non-prescription drugs:** The simultaneous use of prescription drug with non-prescription drugs (e.g. antacids decongestants, aspirin).
2. **Multiple pharmacological effects:** Many drugs used in the therapy have an action on many physiologic systems of body. Therefore, when two drugs are administered simultaneously it can affect some of the same systems.
3. **Multiple physicians:** The patient in a short period visits more than one physician which may result in drug interactions.
4. **Patient – Non-compliance:** Many times patients do not follow the instructions of physician or pharmacist (or patients do not receive the instructions properly regarding medication).
5. **Drug abuse:** There is a tendency of some patients to abuse or misuse the drugs for quick results, causing drug interactions.

Mechanisms of Drug Interactions

The mechanisms of drug interactions are classified as:

(a) Pharmacokinetic drug interactions,

(b) Pharmacodynamic drug interactions, and

(c) Miscellaneous drug interactions.

(A) PHARMACOKINETIC DRUG INTERACTIONS

In these, one drug affects the absorption, distribution, metabolism and excretion (ADME) of another drug resulting in a change of concentration of other drug in plasma.

(I) Interactions affecting gastrointestinal absorption

Different mechanisms affect the gastrointestinal absorption of a drug. The amount of drug absorbed may be reduced or delayed which decreases the drug plasma concentration level, reducing the therapeutic effect. Sometimes the slower absorption rate prolongs the effect of drug causing difficulty as in case of hypnotics. Following are the factors which affects the GI absorption.

(i) pH: The pH of the GI contents affects the absorption of drugs. The non-ionised form of drug (the more lipid soluble) gets absorbed more readily than the ionised form of drug. The acidic drugs remain in the non-ionised form in the stomach (low pH), hence these will get readily absorbed. If antacid is administered with acidic drugs, it will raise the pH of GI contents and inhibits the absorption of the drug.

The enteric coated bisocodyl (oral dosage form of laxative) should not be given with antacid or milk because increase in pH of GI contents may cause disintegration of enteric coating, releasing the drug in stomach causing irritation and vomitting.

(ii) Complexation: Drugs like tetracycline form complexes with metal ions such as calcium, magnesium, aluminium and iron which are poorly absorbed. Hence tetracycline should not be administered alongwith milk (containing calcium) and drugs containing metal ions such as iron containing preparations and antacids.

For example, fluoroquinolones like ciprofloxacin norfloxacin should not be administered with aluminium and magnesium containing antacids since these metal ions complex the fluoroquinolones.

(iii) Adsorption: Antidiarrhoeal mixtures contain the adsorbents like kaolin which adsorb the other medications if administered simultaneously, this decreases the absorption of the medication administered.

(iv) Changes in GI motility: Drugs like cathartics increase the GI motility, resulting in a decreased absorption of drugs which are normally absorbed slowly and which require prolonged contact with absorbing surface.

Anticholinergic drugs decrease GI motility, resulting in increased absorption of drug. The effect may be decreased absorption of drug due to slow dissolution of drug.

Barbiturates are known to reduce the absorption of other drugs. The absorption of warfarin is inhibited by heptabarbitone and that of griseofulvin by phenobarbitone.

Cholestyramine inhibits the GI absorption of acetaminophen. Absorption of digoxin is decreased due to presence of metoclopramide which increases GI motility.

(v) Food: Presence of food in stomach influences the absorption of a number of drugs. Food also reduces the absorption of drug by binding with it, or by changing the pH of GI contents and it reduces the dissolution rate of drug.

The absorption of antibiotics is reduced in presence of food. Hence, penicillin and tetracycline derivatives should be given 1 hour before meal or 2 hours after meal to achieve optimum absorption.

Some drugs such as diazepam achieve higher serum level following food whereas drug like cimetidine needs slower absorption, hence it is advantageous to take it with meal.

(vi) Inhibition of GI enzymes: The absorption of certain drugs depends on their metabolism by the enzymes. If these enzymes are inhibited then the absorption of drugs also decreases.

For example: *Folic acid* - Phenytoin interaction.

Phenytoin inhibits the intestinal enzyme conjugate which is responsible for conversion of poorly absorbed form of folic acid i.e. polyglutamate to readily absorbed form of folic acid i.e. monoglutamate. This results in deficiency of folic acid (Anemia).

(II) Interactions Affecting Distribution of Drugs

The drug gets distributed by binding to plasma proteins. Hence, when two drugs capable of binding to proteins are administered concurrently, the interaction affects the distribution. The drug with greater affinity for binding sites will displace the other from plasma or tissue proteins.

Examples:

(1) Phenyl butazone replaces tolbutamide from protein binding and enhances hypoglycemic effect.

(2) Phenyl butazone displaces the warfarin from its binding sites resulting in the increased amount of free form of warfarin causing haemorrhage.

(III) Interactions Affecting Metabolism of Drugs

(a) Inhibition of metabolism:

(i) Isoniazid inhibits the hydroxylation of diphenyl hydantoin and may cause toxicity of diphenyl hydantoin.

(ii) Cimetidine inhibits the metabolism of benzodiazepines (diazepam) and enhances the sedative effect of these.

(iii) Erythromycin inhibits the hepatic metabolism of carbamazepine increasing its toxicity.

(iv) The enzyme xanthine oxidase (responsible for metabolism of mercaptopurine) is inhibited by Allopurinol, reducing the production of uric acid.

(b) Induction of metabolism:

Barbiturates stimulate the microsomal enzyme system in liver and thus increase metabolic degradation of other drugs such as alcohol, coumarin anticoagulants, phenytoin etc.

(IV) Interactions Affecting Excretion

One drug may block the renal excretion of another by competing for the same tubular transport system or may increase the excretion of the drug by increasing, its ionisation.

(i) Inhibition of excretion: Probenecid competes with penicillin in renal secretion and this inhibits the excretion of penicillin, thus increasing its activity.

Probenecid also decreases the renal excretion of methotrexate and clofibrate.

Quinidine and verapamil both cause increase in the serum digoxin level by inhibiting the renal tubular secretion and renal excretion and non-renal clearance of digoxin.

(ii) Increase in renal excretion: Antacids like sodium bicarbonate make the urine alkaline and thus enhance the ionization of weak acidic drugs like salicyclates, barbiturates and lead to their rapid excretion.

(B) PHARMACODYNAMIC DRUG INTERACTIONS

This involves interaction at pharmacodynamic level of the drug. There may be direct interaction between the drugs or drug effects or interaction at receptor level. This may enhance or inhibit the total effect.

(i) Interaction enhancing the effect: e.g. synergistic effect of trimethoprim and sulphamethoxazole. MAOI and sympathomimetics enhance sympathetic activity.

(ii) Interactions inhibiting the effect: e.g. Acetylcholine and atropine by competitive antagonism oppose the actions of each other.

Alcohol and amphetamine have opposite effects on CNS.

(C) MISCELLANEOUS DRUG INTERACTIONS

(i) Interactions causing electrolyte disturbances: Administration of calcium enhances digitalis toxicity. Similarly thiazide diuretics cause hypokalemia and may enhance digitalis toxicity.

(ii) Wood-Drug Interactions: Tyramine present in food like cheese and banana may not be metabolised by MAO if MAOI is given and a severe hypertensive crisis may result.

(iii) Interactions with formulation additives: e.g. Enteric coated tablet may dissolve in the stomach if antacids are administered concurrently. Additives like CMC and gelatin increase the viscosity around the drug particle, hence, dissolution of the drug decreases.

DRUG-DRUG INTERACTIONS

(A) Analgesic Drug Interactions

The following drugs interact with analgesic drug such as *aspirin*.

Interacting drug	Mechanism of interaction	Significance
1. Alcohol	Aspirin damages the mucosa of stomach causing bleeding that results in excessive faecal blood loss.	Combination of aspirin and alcohol must be avoided.
2. Anticoagulant e.g. *Heparin* *Warfarin* *Dicoumarol*	Aspirin potentiates anti-coagulant activity by displacing coumarins from binding sites and reducing plasma prothrombin. It also decreases platelet adhesiveness and causes gastric mucosal bleeding.	Aspirin should be avoided by patients on oral anti-coagulant therapy.
3. Corticosteroids	Corticosteroids decreases the blood aspirin level by increasing GFR. When steroid dose is reduced it causes increase in blood aspirin which results in salicylism.	Patients should be observed for symptoms of salicylism while stopping the steroids.
4. Insulin and oral hypoglycemic agents	Aspirin displaces tolbutamide and chloropropamide from binding sites and thus decreases insulin requirements.	Aspirin causes profound hypoglycaemia in patients on sulphonylurea drugs.
5. Phenylbutazone	Phenylbutazone inhibits the uricosuric effect of aspirin. Aspirin also competes with phenylbutazone for plasma protein binding.	Physician should be aware of this interaction while treating patients of gouty arthritis.
6. Probenecid	Aspirin inhibits the uricosuric action of probenecid.	Aspirin should not be taken during treatment of gout with - probenecid.
7. PABA (Para-aminobenzoic acid)	PABA blocks the formation of salicyluric acid from salicylic acid causing increased blood salicylate level.	Blood salicylate level increases by PABA.

Interacting drug	Mechanism of interaction	Significance
8. Sulphinpyrazone	Aspirin inhibits the uricosuric action of sulphinpyrazone.	Aspirin and sulphin- pyrazone should not be combined while treating gout.
9. Sulphonamide	The effect of sulphonamides may be enhanced by displacement from protein binding by aspirin.	No clinical problem but it may increase the potency and decrease the duration of action, of sulphonamide.
10. IUDs	The inflammatory activity of IUD may be inhibited by aspirin if used chronically.	Women using IUD should use another form of contraception. Chronic use of aspirin increases the IUD failure rate.

(B) Diuretic drug interactions

Combination	Mechanism of interaction	Significance
1. Diuretic - Anti-diabetic agent	Diuretic increase blood sugar level in diabetics. Due to excessive K^+ loss by diuretic, thiazides and chlorthalidone inhibit the action of antidiabetic drug. Diuretics also cause depression of Islets of Langerhans.	Diabetic patient should be monitored be substituting less diabetogenic diuretic and supplement of potassium.
2. Diuretic – Anti-hypertensive agent	Thiazides increase the hypotensive effect of anti-hypertensives such as guanethedine, ethyl doparauwolfia alkaloids and ganglion blocking agents.	The combination of thiazide and antihypertensive drug is valuable but patient should be watched for excessive hypotension.
3. K^+ – loosing diuretic – cardiac glycoside	The effect and toxicity of cardiac glycosides (Digitalis) are enhanced by hypokalemia caused due to K^+ loosing diuretics.	Replacement K^+ therapy is advisable.
4. Diuretic – corticosteroid	This combination may increase the total K^+ – loss.	Severe K^+ loss disturbs electrolyte balance which must be carefully monitored.
5. Diuretic – Quinidine – Amphetamine – Ephedrine	Acetazolamide and thiazides make the urine alkaline that results in increased renal tubular absorption of Quinidine amphetamine and ephedrine enhancing their side effects and toxicity.	Patients on quinidine should be carefully prescribed with urine alkalinisers ($NaHCO_3$).

Combination	Mechanism of interaction	Significance
6. Thiazides – Alcohol	The vasodilator effects of alcohol may enhance the hypotensive effect of thiazides.	Avoid alcohol.
7. Acetazolamide – Lithium carbonate	Acetazolamide inhibits proximal tubular reabsorption of lithium ions causing its excretion. This could impair the antipsychotic effect.	Avoid this combination or if required increase dose of lithium to compensate its excretion.
8. Ethacrynic acid – Aminoglycoside antibiotic	Ethacrynic acid is ototoxic in its own and will increase the ototoxicity of aminologycoside antibiotic.	Avoid this combination. Alternative diuretic should be substituted.
9. Spironolactone Potassium chloride	Spironolactone conserves potassium and hyperkalemia may result if potassium supplements are also given.	This combination is useful in treating severe potassium depletion. However patient must be monitored for detection of hyperkalemia.
10. Ethacrynic acid – Anticoagulant	Ethacrynic - acid displaces warfarin from plasma binding sites.	Reduction in dose of anticoagulant is necessary.

(C) Cardio-vascular Drug Interactions

(1) Anti-arrhythmic Drug Interactions:

Combination	Mechanism of interaction	Significance
1. Procainamide -Sulphonamide	The antibacterial action of sulphonamide is antagonized by PABA and compounds derived from it, especially procaine and related compounds.	These should not be given concomitantly.
2. Procainamide - cholinergic agents	Procainamide antagonise the effect of cholinergic drugs on skeletal muscles.	Avoid procainamide in myasthenic patients. Quinidine cannot be substituted.
3. Procainamide - antihypertensive agent.	Additive hypotensive effect may occur especially with I.V. or I.M. procainamide.	Possible additive hypotensive effect should be watched.
4. Quinidine - Acetazoliamide	Discussed under diuretic drug interactions.	
5. Quinidine - Cimetidine	Cimetidine inhibit the hepatic metabolism of quinidine.	Cimetidine should be used carefully with patients on quinidine.

(2) Antihypertensive Drug Interactions:

Combination	Mechanism of interaction	Significance
1. Guanethidine – Antidepressants MAOIs.	MAOIs may antazgonise the effects of guanethidine bethanidine.	Difficult to achieve control of hypertension.
2. Methyldopa-antidepressant (MAOIs)	The hypotensive effect of methyl dopa may be diminished by MAOI antidepressants.	Concomitant treatment should be avoided. Hypertension may result.
3. Methyldopa-Ephedrine	Ephedrine has adrenergic action which is inhibited by reducing the amount of noradrenaline available for release.	The local mydriatic effect of ephedrine may be reduced by methyldopa.
4. Methyldopa Sympathomimetic amines	Amphetamine and sympatho-mimetics reduce the hypotensive effect of methyldopa.	Concomitant administration should be followed with care.
5. Reserpine – Ephedrine	Ephedrine was found effective in patients with nasal congestion, drowsiness and depression induced by reserpine therapy.	The combination is clinically useful.
6. Reserpine – Atropine sulphate	The side effects of Reserpine such as nasal congestion can be relieved by atropine.	The combination is clinically useful.
7. Reserpine – Levodopa	The hypotensive and CNS depressant effects of reserpine are enhanced by levodopa. Reserpine decreases the effects of levodopa by causing dopamine depletion in brain.	Avoid this combination Guanethidine and methyldopa also decreases the effects of levodopa. Hence these cannot be substituted in place of reserpine.
8. Propranolol – Insulin	Beta-adrenergic blockade reduces the rise in blood sugar to adrenaline. Propranolol blunts the rebound of blood sugar following insulin-induced hypoglycaemia. It also blocks the clinical signs of hypoglycaemia.	Combination should be used with caution.
9. Propranolol – Digiyalis glycosides.	Propranolol reduces the ventricular rate in auricular fibrillation and flutter effectively with digitalis. Propranolol is also effective in controlling arrhythmias associated with digitalis intoxication.	Arrhythmias which are not controlled by digitalis alone can be effectively controlled by using propranolol in combination.
10. Propranolol – Antidepressant (MAOIs)	MAOIs are contradicated with propranolol since it may result in a severe hypertension.	Although theoretical but nevertheless a dangerous interaction.

(3) Cardiac glycosides Interaction:

Combination	Mechanism of interaction	Significance
1. Cardiac glycosides − Calcium salts	The positive inotropic effect of digitalis is inhibited by higher concentration of calcium resulting in toxicity. Calcium also causes dangerous increase in ATP-ase inhibition.	Injections of calcium salts should not be given during digitalis therapy.
2. Cardiac glycoside – Barbiturate – Phenytoin – Phenyl butazone	Barbiturates, phenytoin and phenyl butazone enhance the rate of metabolism of digitoxin to digoxin through microsomal enzymes.	Avoid these and aware of reduced efficacy of digitoxin.
3. Cardiac glycoside – Sympathomimetics	Combination causes increased liability to ectopic pacemaker activity. Ephedrine enhances the possibility of arrhythmia.	Patients on digitalis therapy should be given sympathomimetic drugs with caution.

(4) Anticoagulant Drug Interaction:

Combination	Mechanism of interaction	Significance
1. Anticoagulant – Analgesic drug	Explained earlier.	Explained earlier.
2. Anticoagulant – Antacid drug	Antacids may cause impaired absorption of coumarins due to alkaline environment which causes ionisation.	Minor effect.
3. Anticoagulant – Chloramphenicol	Chloramphenicol enhances the action of anticoagulant by: (i) Inhibition of coumarin metabolism in liver and (ii) Impairment of absorption of vitamin K from the gut.	Use an alternative antibiotic.
4. Anticoagulant – Penicillin	Penicillin antagonize the anticoagulant effect of heparin.	Be aware of this combination.
5. Anticoagulant – Neomycin – Streptomycin – Tetracyclines – Sulphonamides	These drugs potentiate the anticoagulant effect by reducing the amount of vitamin K synthesized by intestinal flora. Sulphonamides also displaces coumarins from protein binding sites and thus potentiates anticoagulant effect.	These antibiotics should be given with caution to patients on oral anticoagulant therapy.

Combination	Mechanism of interaction	Significance
6. Anticoagulant – Antidepressant MAOIs	MAOIs potentiate the anticoagulant effect of coumarin and may cause haemorrhage.	Avoid this combination.
7. Anticoagulant – Diuretic (Ethacrynic acid)	Explained earlier.	
8. Anticoagulant – Liquid paraffin (Laxative)	Liquid paraffin (used as laxative) decreases the intestinal absorption of lipid-soluble materials (Vitamin K) and thus enhances the oral anticoagulant effect.	Alternative laxative should be recommended whenever prolonged use is necessary.

(D) Gastrointestinal Agents Interactions

Combination	Mechanism of interaction	Significance
1. Anthelmintic – Alcohol	The effective anthelmintic, tetrachloroethylene is slightly absorbed from G.I.T. but in presence of alcohol its absorption increases. This causes CNS depressant side effects and liver toxicity.	Alcohol should not be taken during the anthelmintic treatment.
2. Liquid paraffin (laxative) – Anticoagulant	Explained earlier.	
3. Appetite suppressant e.g. *Amphetamine sulphate*	The appetite suppressants have sympathomimetic activity. In combination with MAOI antidepressants it may cause severe hypertension and hyperpyrexia.	The appetite suppressants should not be given to patients on MAOI drug or within 2 weeks of stopping such drugs.
4. Antacid – Anticoagulant	Explained earlier.	
5. Antacid-Aspirin	Antacid reduces GIT irritation.	Less irritation and better absorption of aspirin.
6. Digoxin – Pectolin mixture	Adsorption of digoxin.	Absorption of digoxin decreases.
7. Cathartics – Slowly absorbed drugs.	Cathartics increases GI motility and moves the drugs fastly through GIT.	Decrease in the rate of absorption of slowly absorbed drugs.
8. Antacid = Cimetidin	Antacid inhibits the absorption of cimetidine and ranitidine.	Separate doses of cimetidine and antacids should be administered.

(E) Hypoglycaemic Drug Interactions

Combination	Mechanism of interaction	Significance
1. Antidiabetic agent – Alcohol	There is a risk of severe hypoglycaemia due to hypoglycaemic effect of alcohol.	Avoid the use of sulphonylureas in alcoholics.
2. Insulin and oral hypoglycemic agents – Aspirin	Aspirin displaces tolbutamide and chlorpropamide from plasma protein binding. The insulin requirements of diabetics can also be reduced by aspirin.	Aspirin causes hypoglycaemia in patients on sulphonylureas.
3. Antidiabetic agent – Anticoagulant	Dicoumarol increases the half-life of tolbutamide in diabetics.	Reduction in dose of sulphonylureas is desirable.
4. Tolbutamide – Chloramphenicol	Chloramphenicol increases the half life of tolbutamide three times.	Alternative antiobiotic should be prescribed.
5. Antidiabetic agent – Sulphonamide	Hypoglycemic action of tolbutamide is enhanced with sulfisoxazole. The half life and serum levels of tolbutamide are also increased. Sulphaphenazole inhibits carboxylation of tolbutamide.	Combination causes hypoglycaemia hence dose of sulphonylurea may have to be reduced.
6. Antidiabetic agent – Anti-inflammatory agent	Phenylbutazone by inhibiting the metabolism and protein binding sulphonylureas, enhances the hypoglycemic effect.	Combination should be avoided, since control of blood sugar is difficult.
7. Antidiabetic agent-β-blocker e.g. *Propranolol*	Propranolol precipitates hypoglycaemia in insulin dependent diabetics. It may be due to blockade of release of glucose from liver.	β-blocker should be given cautiously to patients on anti-diabetic agent.
8. Antidiabetic agent – Thyroid hormone.	Thyroid hormones raise the blood sugar level and cause instability of patients receiving anti-diabetic agent.	Patient should be under careful observation on initiation of thyroid treatment.
9. Antidiabetic agent – Diuretic e.g. *Thiazides, Frusemide, Ethacrynic acid*	These diuretics cause increase in blood sugar level in diabetics. It may be due to K^+ loss.	Monitor patient for decreased diabetic control by substituting less diabetogenic diuretic.

DRUG-FOOD INTERACTIONS

The interaction between MAOI antidepressants and tyramine containing food especially cheese is the best example of drug-food interaction. MAO is an enzyme abundantly present in liver and other tissues. It causes metabolism of serotonin (5-hydroxytryptamine), tyramine and to a lesser extent noradrenaline. Whenever the action of MAO is inhibited, the concentration of serotonin, tyramine and noradrenaline increases, in central nervous system. This causes sudden hypertension and severe headache.

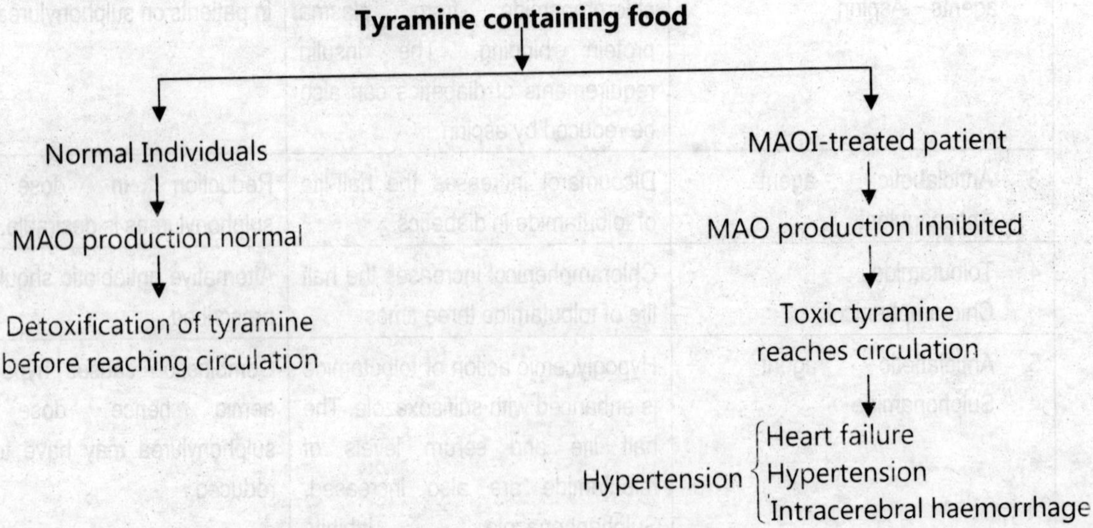

Hence, tyramine containing foods such as cheese, banana, some beers, yeast products and caffeine containing drinks are forbidden to patients on MAO inhibitor therapy due to their dopamine, tyramine or serotonin content.

Some important drug-food interactions are given below.

Name of drug	Type of food	Effect
1. MAOIs	Food rich in tyramine e.g. *Cheese, Banana.*	Hypertensive crisis.
2. Erythromycin	Acidic fruits	Decomposition of drug reducing the effect.
3. Quinidine	Basic foods e.g. *milk, most vegetables*	Decreased renal clearance due to alkalinity of urine.
4. Digoxin Tetracycline	Milk	Reduced GI absorption.
5. Antihypertensives diuretics	Liquorice	Sodium retension, hypokalemia and increased B.P.
6. Griseofulvin	Fatty food	Increased absorption rate.
7. Anticoagulant	Food rich in vitamin K e.g. egg, yolk, green, leafy vegetables.	Vitamin K enhances the synthesis of clotting factors in liver decreasing anticoagulant effect of drug.

Vitamin Interactions:

Combination	Mechanism of interaction	Significance
1. Vitamin A – Mineral oil	Mineral oil may impair the GI absorption of vitamin A.	Separate the doses of mineral oil and vitamin A to avoid the mixing in GIT.
2. Pyridoxine – Barbiturate	Pyridoxine enhances the metabolism of barbiturates.	Special precaution is not necessary.
3. Pyridoxine – Levodopa	Pyridoxine enhance the metabolism of levodopa thus decreasing the amount available at the site of action in the brain.	Combination should be avoided.
4. Vitamin B_{12} – Chloramphenicol	Chloramphenicol interferes with the maturation of erythrocytes in patients on vitamin B_{12} therapy.	Alternative antibiotic should be used.
5. Vitamin E – Oral anticoagulant	Vitamin E may interfere with the effect of vitamin K in the production of clotting factors.	Combination should be avoided.
6. Vitamin K – Oral anticoagulant	(1) Vitamin K could offset oral anticoagulant induced depression of clotting factor synthesis. (2) Delay in absorption of warfarin caused by food (leafy vegetables).	Patient should be warned to avoid sudden increase in the diet.
7. Vitamin D – Anticonvulsant (Phenytoin Phenobarbital)	Anticonvulsant stimulates the metabolism of vitamin D that results in lowered blood calcium level, causing rickets.	Calcium rich diet is beneficial. Exposure of patient to sunlight is advised.
8. Vitamins – Oral contraceptives	Oral contraceptives inhibit the gastric enzymes required for absorption of these vitamins resulting in their deficiency.	Supplement of vitamins is advised.

QUESTIONS

1. Define "drug interaction". Classify the mechanisms of drug interactions.
2. Describe with examples pharmacokinetic drug interactions.
3. Describe with examples pharmacodynamic drug interactions.
4. Give two combinations of antihypertensive drug interactions which are clinically useful.
5. Give two combinations with mechanism of interaction and significance of the following:
   (a) Analgesic drugs.
   (b) Antihypertensive drugs.
   (c) Anticoagulant drugs.
6. Give the mechanism of interaction and clinical significance of the following drug combinations:
   (i) Propranolol - digitalis glycosides.
   (ii) Diuretic - antidiabetic agent.
   (iii) Reserpine - ephedrine.
   (iv) Anticoagulant - antibiotic.
7. Write in short about drug-food interaction.
8. Give the causes of drug interactions and describe its various sites.
9. Describe the factors which affect the GI absorption of a drug.

***

7

ADVERSE DRUG REACTIONS

Many definitions of the term 'adverse drug reaction' have been given over the past years. The one which is most valuable is that which emphasizes the patient's viewpoint – "Any undesired or unintended effect of drug treatment."

Drugs may interact in many different ways and the resulting effects may be beneficial or adverse. The beneficial drug reactions are used to minimise the risks of a particular form of therapy or to improve its effectiveness.

For example, carbidopa is used in combination with L-dopa to minimise systemic effects of latter while maximising the dose absorbed into CNS. Sulphonamide is used in combination with antifolate drug to improve the effectiveness. e.g. cotrimoxazole combination of oestrogen-progestogen drug as one type of hormonal contraceptive.

Adverse drug reactions (ADRs) have been defined by the World Health Organization as "Any response to a drug which is noxious and unintended, and which occurs at doses used in man for prophylaxis, diagnosis or therapy."

Classification of Adverse Drug Reactions

Many factors are responsible for the etiology of adverse drug reactions. These reactions are classified as :

(1) Excessive pharmacological effect

(2) Secondary pharmacological effect

(3) Idiosyncrasy

(4) Allergic drug reactions

(5) Genetically determined toxicity

(6) Toxicity following drug withdrawal.

(1) Excessive Pharmacological Effect

It is common experience of patients receiving CNS depressants, cardioactive, hypotensive and hypoglycaemic agents. If excessive dose is given, all patients are at risk of developing this reaction. Certain patients are more susceptible to this reaction even when an average dose is prescribed which includes:

(a) Patients with kidney disease who hive lost more than 70% of their kidney function.

(b) Patients with hypoalbuminemia due to failure of albumin production by liver or excessive loss of albumin as in nephrotic syndrome.

(c) Patient's age: Neonates, infants and elderly patients. The detailed knowledge of pharmacokinetic behaviour of administered drug is necessary for dosage adjustment to minimise the risks of excessive pharmacologic effect.

(2) Secondary Pharmacological Effects

Many drugs have several pharmacological actions at an average dose, yet they are prescribed solely for one of these actions. For example, antihistamines are frequently prescribed for allergic skin reactions or for their anti-nausea effects. It has concomitant effect of drowsiness and if given to a commercial traveller, a bus driver it can have disastrous consequences. These secondary pharmacological effects often involve CNS depression which may be dangerous if patients are also consuming hypnotics, tranquillizers or OTC medications. Thus alongwith excessive pharmacological effects, secondary pharmacological effects provide a large bulk of undesired drug effects experienced by patients.

(3) Indiosyncracy

This term is primarily used for unusual, unexpected drug effects. It also includes drug induced foetal abnormalities, such as phocomelia developing in offsprings of mothers exposed to thalidomide. Although thalidomide has a powerful potential as a teratogen, the mechanism whereby it exerts this potential is unknown. If it is given to mothers during the initial period of gestation when the limb buds are forming, it results into sealed limbs.

Another indiosyncratic reaction is drug induced cancer. Because of long induction period between exposure to drug and development of tumours little is known about drug factors in the etiology of cancer. It is found that use of following drugs may cause the cancer of specific organ.

Cancer of Organ	Causative drug
Vaginal adenocarcinorna	High doses of stilboestrol during pregnancy.
Kidney pelvis	Analgesic induced nephropathy
Uterus	Oestrogens (Long-term)
Lymphoid tissue	Azathioprine, cyclophosphamide (long-term use)

(4) Allergic drug reactions

These reactions are common but unpredictable in their occurrence. It ranges from very mild skin reactions to major anaphylaxis and sometimes death. The term "allergy" is used to indicate an immunological reaction. Another term "hypersensitivity" is synonymous with allergy.

An allergic reaction due to drug allergy depends upon the following factors:

(a) The reaction does not resemble the expected pharmacological activity of the drug.

(b) There is delay between initial exposure to drug and development of allergic reaction.

(c) Reaction recurs on repeated exposure even to traces of the allergenic drug.

To elicit an allergic reaction, a drug (or its metabolite) must act as antigen which reacts with the antibodies by linking with circulating macromolecules. It then releases the active peptides such as serotonin, kinins, prostaglandins and histamine at various body sites causing the allergic reaction. Sometimes the blocking antibodies are produced, usually IgG, IgM, which combine with the antigen before the more specific reactor antibodies can reach it. Another possibility is that free drug or its metabolite may fix onto binding sites on antibodies before the drug-macromolecule (antigen) complex has been formed in large quantities.

Once antibodies are formed, the reaction may be generalised or localised to specific tissues, and the symptoms of drug allergy depends upon which of the above mechanisms contribute to the response. Allergic drug reactions seen in human and the causative drugs are given below.

Allergic reaction	Causative drugs
Anaphylaxis	Penicillins, anaesthetics, dextrans. Iodine containing compounds.
Skin rashes	Sulphonamides, penicillins, barbiturates.
Haemolytic anemias	Sulphonamides, penicillins, quinidine, methyldopa.
Hepatitis	Phenothiazines, methyldopa.
Leucopenia	Sulphonamides, thiouracils phenylbutazone.
Thrombocytopenia	Quinidine, thiazides, digoxin thiouracils.
Nephritis	Methicillin, oxacillin, nafcillin.

Anaphylaxis is most serious of allergic reactions and is usually due to IgE activity. It may be generalized or localized to gut giving abdominal pain and diarrhoea, bronchi giving asthma or skin giving oedema. In generalized anaphylaxis, a circulatory collapse with hypotension, bronchospasm and skin rash occurs. It is due to release of peptides into circulation and can be counteracted by rapid administration of adrenaline for immediate effect.

(5) Genetically determined Toxicities

Patients of selected genetic make-up are at greater risks for specific drug toxicities e.g. patients with porphyria are uniquely susceptible to CNS depressing effects of barbiturates. Due to individual variations, the ability to acetylate the drugs in the liver is highly variable. Some patients are "slow" acetylators while others are 'rapid' acetylators. Slow acetylators of drugs such as procainamide, isoniazid are at greater risk of developing toxicity than fast acetylators. 60% of Britains and 70% of Jews are slow acetylators while only 10% of Japanese and Chinese are slow acetylators.

Patients with pseudocholinesterase deficiency (heriditary disorder) are highly susceptible to succinylcholine.

Individuals with deficiency of glucose – 6-phosphate dehydrogenase enzyme involved in the degradation of glucose by pentose-phosphate pathway are at more risk of developing haemolysis after use of antimalarial drugs primaquine, aminoquindline sulphoxiamides etc. Following are the genetically determined types of drug toxicities.

Hereditary Condition	Drugs Causing Toxicity
1. Pseudocholinesterase deficiency	Succinyl choline
2. Porphyria	Barbiturates, sulphonamides
3. Glucose-6-phosphate dehydrogenase deficiency	Antimalarials, quinidine, nitrofurantoin, sulphas
4. Glaucoma	Corticosteroids
5. Methaemoglobinemia	Phenacetin, salicylates

(6) Toxicity following Drug Withdrawal

After long term use of many medications, tolerance is developed at cellular level. Sudden withdrawal of such medications may give rise to severe adverse effects. It happens usually with drugs acting on CNS such as narcotic analgesics, hypnotics, ethyl alcohol but also happens with some hypotensive agents (Clonidine) and corticosteroids.

Clonidine is a mild hypotensive agent which has the property of causing severe rebound hyptertension if its use is discontinued suddenly.

Long-term use of corticosteroids results in the atrophy of recepient's adrenal glands. Sudden withdrawal of these can therefore causes acute adrenal crisis (Addison's disease). This is avoided by gradual removal of corticosteroids over a period of weeks depending on length of time these have been consumed.

Causes of Adverse Drug Reactions

Many factors are responsible for the adverse effects of drugs on patients receiving them. The adverse effects of the drug depends on its dose, duration, toxicity and other individual factors such as sex, age, genetics, compliance of patient and total number of drugs administered.

Whether a patient experiences the toxicity of drug depends on its dose.

The pharmacokinetics of the drug may also affect the drug toxicity. Alteration in pharmacokinetics of drug may result in abnormally higher concentration of drug at receptor site, resulting in adverse effect.

Therapeutic index of a drug is also responsible for the adverse effects. The drug with small therapeutic index is more prone to produce adverse effects than with large therapeutic index e.g. Therapeutic index of amphotericin B is small while that of acetaminophen is large. Hence 75% of patients receiving amphotericin B show the adverse effects while less than 1% of patients receiving acetaminophen show the adverse effects.

Age: Infants are more prone to adverse effects because of incomplete development of liver enzyme system. Also elderly patients show higher incidence of adverse effects.

Heredity: Discussed previously.

Poor patient compliance can also cause excessive dose of the drug.

Methods of Detecting Adverse Drug Effects

The common cause of drug induced disease is the excessive pharmacological effects of drugs. Thus is readily predictable. There are some other types of drug induced diseases which are more difficult to detect and quantitiate (Non-predictable). The various methods are given as follows.

(1) Spontaneous case reports: It is common method of arousing suspicion about drug related diseases. A prescriber suspects that a condition arising in a patient may be drug related. He therefore reports either in a letter to the medical journals or to the manufacturer of drug. By this means other prescribers are alerted to the possibility of drug-disease relationship. "Spontaneous Reporting Agencies" are set up to collect and colate such case reports. Although the resulting information collected gives no idea of the frequency with which a given event is caused by a drug, it indicates that a number of prescribers feel that the event is possibly drug-related.

(2) Vital statistics and record linkage studies: The details of cause of death (as recorded on death certificate) or of hospitalization (as recorded on the discharge letter) are routinely collected and analysed. It gives early warning of an epidemic of drug-related disease. Record linkage studies can be used to great effect in the search for drug-induced disease.

(3) Cohort studies: The 'Cohort' means identifying a group of recipients of a drug of interest and observing these patients for varying lengths of time and recording what happens to them. This type of study is used for short term clinical trial of a new drug. Cohort studies involving long term clinical trials are more difficult to organize. Thus, this method is of great value for detecting predictable adverse effects due to excessive pharmacological effects arising during or immediately after short term treatment.

(4) Case-control studies: It involves the comparison of group of patients with a disease which is thought to be due to a drug (the 'cases') with a group of patients who do not have the disease (the 'controls'). The drug histories of the cases and controls are obtained and compared. If a drug is causing the disease then its use amongst the cases will be far in excess of that found in the controls. Case control studies can, be conducted rapidly and efficiently at relatively low cost. However, it must be conducted correctly and resulting data must be interpreted correctly.

Typical features of the method are:

(a) The cases must be selected carefully. The disease must be defined clearly, precisely and accurately. The disease under study must have reasonable risk of being drug-induced.

(b) The controls obtained should be from similar population of cases with the exception that controls do not have the disease of interest. Controls are usually hospitalized patients. They should not include patients admitted for conditions which are indications of drug of interest or which are caused or prevented by the drug of interest.

(c) The method used to describe drug use must be identical in cases and controls.

(d) Interpretation of results must be accurate.

Drug Induced Diseases

At times drugs used to cure one disease may induce another disease condition on various organs of the body.

(1) Drug Induced Haematologic Disorders

The establishment of American Medical Association (AMA) committee on blood dyscrasias was concerned with the incidence of aplastic anemia due to chloramphenicol. The expansion of this committee into a "Registry on Adverse Reactions" takes place in 1961.

Aplastic anemia (Pancytopenia) : The drugs which cause bone marrow aplasia include alkylating agents, antimetabolites, antibiotics, vinca alkaloids. The antibacterial drug, chloramphenicol phenybutazone, oxyphenbutazone and indomethacin are the most common causes of a plastic anemia chloramphenicol causes the bone marrow toxicity in two ways. One is by inhibiting the mitochondrial protein synthesis and the other which is much serious by causing true bone marrow aplasia which cannot be prevented by chloramphenicol withdrawal.

Agranulocytosis: It is another drug induced condition due to destruction of granulocytic leucocytes by the antibodies. This condition may happen due to toxic depression of bone marrow stem cells after prolonged administration of a drug in large doses. Drugs which induce agranulocytosis include sulfonamides, sulfonylureas, phenothiazines antihydroid drugs, phenylbutazone and semisynthetic penicillins, antitubercular drugs.

Thrombocytopenia: The reduction in the count of thrombocytes (Platelets) is due to the bone marrow suppression and the destruction of platelets. The cytotoxic drugs like chloramphenicol, sulphanomides, phenothiazines, antiepileptics causes the bone marrow suppression.

The drugs which form the immune complexes that destroy platelets are quinine, quinidine, aspirin, methyldopa, cardiotonics, acetazolamide.

Haemolytic anemia: The haemolytic anemia may occur due to genetic abnormality or acquired immunological abnormality. Haemolysis occurs in patients with deficiency of glucose-6-phosphate dehydroigenase. The immune haemolytic reaction takes, place with methyldopa, levodopa and mefenamic acid and streptomycin. These drugs bind to the proteins in the R.B.C. and cause haemolysis.

(2) Drug Induced Liver Disorders

The liver is the major site for metabolism and excretion of drugs. The drugs capable of producing liver damage are classified into two categories:

(a) Drugs that directly damage the hepatocytes of the liver due to their chemical structure.

(b) Drugs causing liver damage through host hypersensitivity.

Drugs causing liver damage i.e. hepatotoxins include isoniazid, tetracycline, acetaminophen, iron, metho-trexate and aspirin.

Acetaminophen produces toxic metabolites in liver which is cause liver necrosis. In case of isoniazid, elevation of liver enzymes such as serum glutamic oxaloacetic transaminase (SGOT) takes place.

The hypersensitivity type of reactions are the allergic manifestations causing symptoms like rash, fever, arthralgia and eosinophillia. These reactions are of two types viz. hepatitis like and cholestatic. Cholestatic type of reaction is caused due to chlorpromazine, tricyclic antidepressants, methyldopa, erythromycin, chlorpropamide and tolbutamide.

(3) Drug Induced Gastrointestinal Disorders

Most drugs are taken orally, hence there is maximum possibility of GI disorders. The common adverse drug- reactions include nausea, vomitting, constipation, anorexia, dyspepsia and ulceration. Sometimes GI haemorrhage and pancreatitis may occur.

Adverse Drug Reaction	Causative drug
1. Nausea and vomiting.	Most frequently to all orally administered drug.
2. Dysgensia (Altered taste sensation)	Penicillamine, metronidazole, levodopa, captopril.
3. Dyspepsia and ulceration of gastric mucosa.	All non-steroidal anti-inflammatory drugs (NSAID).
4. Constipation	Morphine, haematinics, Nifedipine, Antihistamines, Vinca alkaloids.
5. GI haemorrhage	Corticosteroids.
6. Ulceration in small intestine	Potassium chloride tablets (Enteric coated).
7. Diarrhoea and colitis	Antibiotics especially lincomycin, chloramphenicol, neomycin and other antibiotics and cholinergics.

(4) Drug Induced Renal Disorders

Since most drugs are excreted through urine, various processes in the kidney and high solute concentration in the renal medulla expose the renal cells to higher concentration of drug causing various adverse effects.

Adverse effect	Causative drug
1. Acute Renal Ischaemia	NSAIDs, captopril.
2. Renal tubular toxicity	Aminoglycoside antibiotics, amphotericin B, cyclosporin A, organic iodides, cisplatin, polymixin.
3. Acute Renal Failure	Quinine, nitrofurantoin triamterene, captopril, NSAIDs.
4. Diabetes insipidus	Lithium, sulphonylureas.
5. Interstitial Nephritis.	
(a) Acute	NSAIDs, sulphonamides, diuretics, synthetic penicillins, cephalosporins
(b) Chronic	Large doses of analgesics
6. Kidney stone	Sulphonamides

The effect of acute renal failure by NSAIDs occur due to inhibition of prostaglandin synthetase by these drugs. This results in vasoconstriction and decreased renal blood flow. The risk becomes greater in patients of CCF, cirrhosis and nephrotic syndrome.

ACE inhibitors like captopril prevent vasconstriction in the efferent arteriole and thus decrease the glomerular filtration rate causing renal failure.

(5) Drug Induced Pulmonary Disorders

The most common drug induced disorders of lungs are bronchoconstriction and asthma. Aspirin and NSAIDs inhibits the prostaglandin synthesis. Penicillin is the most common drug causing allergic bronchoconstriction. The other antibiotics include streptomycin, chloramphenicol, tetracycline and erythromycin. The long term use of Busulfan (Cytotoxic drug for leukemia), Nitrofurantoin and Bleomycin causes the pulmonary toxicity. The symptoms include cough, dyspnoea and fever. Pulmonary fibrosis also occurs.

Drugs such as β-adrenoreceptor agonists and antagonists cause acute asthma.

The excessive dose of aminoglycoside antibiotic causes paralysis of respiratory muscles due to neuromuscular blockade.

(6) Drug Induced Skin Disorders

Skin is the most sensitive organ of the body, hence about one third of all reported adverse drug reactions involve the skin.

Adverse effect	Causative drug
1. Toxic eruptions Alopecia	Bromides, allopurinol, sulphonamides, oral anticoagulants, chloroquine, ampicilin, penicillin G, methyldopa, reserpine.
2. Allergic reactions	
(a) Eczema	Allopurinol, warfarin
(b) Erythema multiformae	Penicillin, barbiturates, salicylates, isoniazid, phenytoin.
(c) Erythema nodosum	Sulphanomides.
(d) Stevens-Johnson syndrome	Sulphonamides, phenobarbital, penicillins, phenytoin
(e) Toxic Epidermal Necrolysis (TEN) or Lyell's syndrome	(a) Phenolphthalein, sulphonamides, allopurinol, gold salts, chromaphenicol.
(f) Hirsutism	Corticosteroid, long-term phenytoin, acetazolamide, Tamoxifen, Minoxidil, oral contraceptives.
(g) Systemic lupus erythematosus	Sulphonamides, griseofulvin, hydralazine.

(7) Drug Induced Ocular Diseases

Every structure of eye get adversely affected by drugs. The anticholinergics and ganglion blocking agents decreases the tear production which is essential for healthy eye. Practolol causes a permanent reduction in tear production causing corneal ulceration.

The most common drugs causing ocular toxicity include phenothiazines, antimalarials i.e. chloroquine, antiarrhythmic amiodarone and corticosteroids.

Adverse effect	Causative drug
1. Corneal ulceration due to decreased tear production.	Practolol anticholinergics Ganglion-blocking agents.
2. Pigmentary retinal damage	Chloroquine, phenothiazines
3. Glaucoma	Atropine, corticosteroids e.g. Betamethasone, anticholinergics.
4. Cataract	Corticosteroids, chlorpromazine.
5. Optic neuritis	Isoniazid, chloramphenicol, sulpha drugs.
6. Amblyopia	Chlorpropamide, Nicotinic acid, Alcohol.

(8) Drug Induced reurotoxicity:

The adverse reactions of drugs causing damage to nervous system are of two types :

(i) Extrapyramidal reactions: These occur due to phenothiazines, reserpine, methyldopa and haloperidol.

(ii) Myasthenia like reactions: These occur due to aminoglycoside antibiotics, trimethadione and colistimethane.

(9) Drug Induced Ototoxicity:

Ototoxicity due to drug is of two types viz. vestibular toxicity and cochlear toxicity affecting the vestibule and cochlea of internal ear respectively. The vestibular toxicity results in impairment of balance of the body whereas the cochlear toxicity results in permanent loss of hearing. The drugs causing vestibular toxicity include streptomycine and minocycline (Tetracycline).

Aminoglycoside antibiotics such as neomycin, streptomycin, gentamycin, amikacin are the most ototoxic drugs causing permanent damage. These drugs destroy the outer hair cells in the spiral organ of corti.

Diuretics such as furosemide and ethacrynic acid also cause ototoxicity in patients with renal failure. Tinnitus and bilateral hearing loss may also occur in patients treated with salicylates. This hearing loss is reversible.

Teratogenicity :

The term "teratogenic" means monster producing (teratos = monster). The administration of certain drugs to pregnant woman, specifically during the first trimester of pregnancy results in foetal abnormalities. Such drugs are called as teratogenic or teratogen. The use of thalidomide as sedative, hypnotic in early 1960s in Germany brought to light the problem of teratogenicity children delivered to mothers on this drug had sealed limbs (phocomelia). Hence now in every country, the FDA requirement is to conduct toxicological studies in preclinical evaluation to detect the potential for a drug to cause birth defects. The risk benefit ratio in every case must be detected and then the decision taken.

For example, phenytoin, an antiepileptic drug has been associated with foetal abnormalities like cleft palate. However the risk to the foetus after withdrawal of a drug may be far greater than risk of developing foetal abnormalities.

Methotrexate (antienoplastic drug) on discontinution may show serious adverse effects for the mother than the risk of developing foetal damage.

Following are the drugs having teratogenic effect:

Sex hormones	–	Androgens, progesterone.
Antiepileptics	–	Phenobarbitone, phenytoin.
Antineoplastic drugs	–	Cyclophosphamide, busulphan, methotrexate, chlorambucil.
Antithyroid drugs	–	Carbimazole, Ethyl alcohol, sulphonylureas, corticosteroids and tobacco smoke.

QUESTIONS

1. Define 'Adverse Drug Reaction'. Classify all the reactions.
2. What are the causes of adverse drug reactions ?
3. Describe various methods of detecting adverse drug effect.
4. Write in brief about :
   (i) Idiosyncrasy
   (ii) Allergic drug reactions
   (iii) Teratogenicity
   (iv) Drug induced liver disorders
   (v) Drug induced haematologic disorders.
5. Name the causative drug and induced disorder of the following organs: Lung, kidney, digestive system and eye.

***

8

TOXICOLOGY

It is a branch of medical science which deals with study of poisons with reference to the following: (i) Sources, (ii) Characters and properties, (iii) Symptoms, (iv) Lethal dose, (v) Remedial measures, (vi) Methods of detection, (vii) Autopsy findings.

It also includes laws regarding their sale and prescription.

A "poison" is defined as any substance which when administered, inhaled or swallowed or applied locally causes deleterious effects on the body. Thus, a medicine in a toxic dose is a poison and a poison in small dose may be a medicine. Hence if any substance is administered with the intention to save life, it is called a medicine and if it is given to cause the harm to the body, it is poison.

Laws Governing the Possession and Sale of Poison

Under the following acts the poison can be purchased, stored and sold.

(i) Poisons Act, 1919.

(ii) Drug Act, 1940.

(iii) Pharmacy Act, 1948,

(iv) Drugs and Magic Remedies (Objectionable Advertisement) Act, 1954.

(v) Narcotic Drugs and Psychotropic substances Act, 1985.

Classification of Poisonous Substances

The purpose of poisoning in case of human beings may be suicidal, homicidal, stupefying or accidental. Depending on the mechanism of action of poisonous substances, these are classified as:

(I) Irritant substances: These are of three types:

(a) Inorganic: (i) Non-metallic – Phosphorus, Chlorine, Bromine, Iodine.

(ii) Metallic – Lead, Mercury, Copper, Zinc, Arsenic, Manganese.

(b) Organic **(i) Animal origin:** Snake, Scorpion, Insects, Cantherides.

(ii) Vegetable origin: Ergot, Aloe, Capsicum, Castor oil seeds, etc.

(c) Mechanical: (i) Powdered glass.

(II) Corrosive Substances: Strong acids and alkalies such as hydrochloric acid, sulphuric acid, carbolic acid, oxalic acid, caustic soda, sodium carbonate, ammonium carbonate etc.

(III) Neurotic (Substances acting on Nervous system)

e.g. (i) Cerebral poisons: opium, sedatives and hypnotics, insecticides, cocaine, hyoscyamus.

(ii) Spinal poisons: Nux vomica.

(iii) Peripheral poisons: curare alkaloids, conium.

(IV) Cardiac (Substances acting on heart)

e.g. Digitallis, stropanthus, aconite, tobacco.

(V) Pulmonary depressants: (Substances acting on lungs) e.g. Gases such as carbonmonoxide, coal gas.

(VII) Miscellaneous: e.g. Analgesics, antipyretics, stimulants, antidepressants, antihistamines, hallucinogens etc.

The poisoning in human beings is of two types:

(a) Acute poisoning and
(b) Chronic poisoning.

(a) Acute poisoning: The symptoms of acute poisoning appear immediately after the ingestion of poison. They increase in severity and may follow death. The poison can be detected in the ingested substance or vomit, stool and urine of the victim. The main symptoms are vomitting and diarrhoea or convulsions and coma.

(b) Chronic poisoning: The symptoms of chronic poisoning appear gradually. The symptoms may disappear after removal of victim from his surrounding. Poison can be detected in the ingested substance or stool, vomit and urine of the victim. The main symptoms are chronic ill-health malaise, repeated attacks of GI irritation, and increased cachexia.

General Treatment of Poisoning: When the poison is known, the specific treatment should be given but when poison is unknown, the treatment should be given on the general basis. The main aim of the treatment is to save the life of the victim by maintaining the respiration and circulation or beating of the heart.

The five basic principles of general treatment of poisoning includes:

(A) To remove unabsorbed poison from the body.
(B) To use antidotes.
(C) To excrete absorbed poison.
(D) To treat the general symptoms of the victim.
(E) To maintain the victims general condition.

(A) To Remove Unabsorbed Poison From the Body

Poison enters the body by different routes. Following measures should be taken for the removal of unabsorbed poison.

(a) Poison entered through nose (Inhalation): When any toxic gas has been inhaled, the victim immediately be taken to place where there is fresh air. Artificial respiration should be given immediately.

(b) Poison entered through contact with skin, eye or wound: Wash out the poison with plain warm water and if specific antidote is available, neutralize the poison with it.

(c) Poison entered through injection: In case of injected poison, the unabsorbed poison may be removed by making incisions at the point of injection and causing it to bleed. With the blood flow, the poison comes out. After this the poison may be removed by suction. The application of tourniquet proximal to the point of injection helps in slowing the absorption of poison.

(d) Poison entered through mouth: The unabsorbed poison nay be removed by inducing vomitting and washing the stomach (gastric lavage).

Vomitting: Emetics are the agents which produce vomitting. Emesis should not be done if the poisoning is by strychnine, corrosives or patient is in coma condition. The common household emetics are mustard powder (15 gm), common salt two-tablespoon, Ipecac 1-2 gm, ammonium carbonate 1-2 gm, Zinc sulphate 1-2 gm in 200 ml water are some other emetics. The dose of 6 mg of Apomorphine by S.C. injection followed by 5-10 mg Naloxon hydrochloride by I.M. or I.V. (to counteract the narcotic effects of apomorphine) is widely used emetic. Apomorphine has following advantages viz.

(i) Quick onset of action i.e. within 5 min.

(ii) It facilitates gastric lavage.

(iii) It produces reflux of upper intestinal contents into the stomach.

The disadvantage of apomorphine is, it should not be used in depressed patients or those in coma condition. Its effect after oral administration is slow.

Vomitting is contraindicated in case of acid or alkali poisoning since it may cause rupture of the stomach.

Gastric lavage (Stomach wash): It is the best method for the removal of unabsorbed poison from the stomach. It is useful only upto 4 to 6 hours after ingestion of poison.

Method: The patient should be prone on one side with the head down. This will help in respiratory drainage and prevent the material entering the respiratory tract. The stomach tube is a flexible rubber tube about 1.5 meter in length, 12.7 mm in external diameter. A filter funnel is provided at upper end, a suction bulb to suck the contents and remove any obstruction in the tube. A mouth gag with a central hole at the level of 50 cm from lower end (to avoid bitting of tube) of tube is provided. The lower end of the tube is perforated. The lower end is lubricated with liquid paraffin or glycerine and passed through the hole in mouth gag down the oesophagus. At the level marked the tip of tube lies in the stomach. Make sure of it and run about 0.5 lit. of plain warm water through funnel which is held above the level of patients mouth. Then lower the funnel below the level of mouth to allow the gastric contents to be removed out. The process is repeated with warm water or fluid containing specific antidote until the returned fluid is of same colour as the lavage fluid. After lavage, some of antidote may remain in the stomach. To remove it and other poison from intestine sodium sulphate or magnesium sulphate solution should be administered to cause purgation. Activated charcoal should be given to absorb alkaloidal poison.

(B) Antidotes

These are the substances which neutralise the effects of poison. When the poison has been absorbed in to the systemic circulation, use of only emesis or lavage is not sufficient. The specific antidote must be administered to counteract the effects of poison. The antidotes are of four types:

(1) Physical antidote

These are substances which inhibit the absorption of poison e.g. Demulcents such as fats, oils and egg albumin. The demulcents form a coat on the mucous membrane of G.I.T. and thus, inhibit the absorption of poison. Fats and oils should not be used as an antidote in phosphorus poisoning since phosphorus is soluble in it. Banana is the best antidote for glass poisoning. Charcoal is used to absorb alkaloidal poison.

(2) Chemical antidote

It is a substance which interacts chemically with a poison to form an insoluble precipitate which is non-toxic or it oxidises the poison to its non-toxic form.

Poison	Antidote
Acids	Magnesium oxide, calcium oxide
Carbonic acid	Magnesium sulphate
Lead	Sulphates of alkalis
Oxalic acid	Lime
Phosphorus	Copper sulphate
Alkaloids	Tannins

(3) Physiological antidote

It is a substance which produces the effect opposite to that of the poison without interacting chemically with it. These are antagonists of poison. Sometimes the antagonism may be incomplete and the antagonists itself may produce an adverse effects.

Poison	Antagonist/Chelator
Morphine	Caffeine, Naloxone
Organophosphorus Compounds	Atropine
Pilocarpine	Atropine
Strychnine	Chloroform
Arsenic	BAL, EDTA
Copper	BAL, Penicillamine
Gold	BAL
Lead	BAL, EDTA, Penicillamine, DMSA
Mercury	BAL, Penicillamine
Thallium	Prussian blue
Iron	Desferrioxamine B.

Chelating agents are substances which produce a firm non-ionized cyclic complex, (called as chelate) with cations. The important chelating agents are BAL, EDTA, Penicillamine and Desferrioxamine-B.

(1) BAL (British anti-lewiste) (Dimercaprol): It is a chelating agent used in the treatment of heavy metal poisoning. The heavy metals have an affinity for thiol (–SH) groups and combine with them in body tissues, displacing the hydrogen and depriving the body of these enzymes whose activities depends on a thiol group. If BAL is administered sufficiently in excess amount, the heavy metals react with it and thus protects the enzyme system of the body. The resultant complex formed is stable and excreted without any damage to liver or kidney. BAL is administered in a dose of 3-5 mg/kg I.M. at the interval of 4 hours for first 2 days, interval of 4-6 hours for additional 2 days and interval of 6-12 hours for additional 7 days.

(2) EDTA (Ethylene Diamine Tetra Acetate): It is a chelating agent which has great affinity for the lead. The chelated lead is excreted in the urine. Short courses of treatment are advised to avoid the depletion of metallic ions essential for metabolism.

Dose: 75 mg/kg 24 hours I.M. or slow I.V. infusion given in 3 to 6 divided doses for 5 days may be repeated for a second course after a minimum interval of 2 days. Each course should not exceed a total of 500 mg/kg.

(3) Penicillamine: It has a stable SH group which confers the chelating action. It is less toxic than EDTA and can be given orally. It is used in copper, lead and mercury poisoning. It is also used for treatment of hepatolenticular degeneration (Wilson's disease).

Dose: 100 mg/kg/day (max. 1 g) in divided doses for upto 5 days. For long term therapy it should not exceed 40 mg/kg/day.

(4) Deferrioxamine: It is a chelating agent which chelates iron in the stomach and binds iron in the blood. Thus it is useful both orally and intravenously for avoiding systemic absorption and removing the absorbed iron.

Dose: Oral 8 - 12 g in 40 to 60 ml distilled water I.V. 2 g in 5% laevulose solution.

[140 mg of Desferrioxamine can bind about 1 g of ferrous sulphate - (200 mg of iron)]

(5) Universal antidote: When the nature of ingested poison is unknown, the universal antidote is used

(i) To neutralise the acids,

(ii) To absorb the alkaloidal poisons, and

(iii) To precipitate or chelate the metals, certain glucosides and alkaloids.

Composition of universal antidote

1. Magnesium - 1 part
2. Activated charcoal - 2 parts
3. Tannic acid - 1 part

The mixture should be given in a dose of 1 tablespoon in 200 ml of water once or twice.

(C) To Excrete Absorbed Poison

After 6 hours of ingestion of poison, emesis and gastric lavage are useless. The poison has entered the intestine and hence the following measures should be taken to excrete the poison through urine and faeces.

1. Forced disuresis: Use I.V. chlorthiazide and/or mannitol.
2. Use of cathartics.

3. Use of hot packs: For increased sweating.
4. Peritoneal dialysis: For salicylate poisoning in children.
5. Haemodialysis: For excretion of barbiturates, salicylates, thiocyanates, bromides.
6. Exchange transfusion is only feasible with small children. All types of poisons are removed by this technique.

(D) To Treat the General Symptoms of the Victim

When the poison is unknown, the symptoms provide the best clue for the treatment.

Symptom	Treatment
Pain	Morphine
Circulation failure	Cardiac Stimulants
Respiratory failure	Artificial respiration
Dehydration	Saline infusion

Addition of glucose and sodium bicarbonate in saline infusion is beneficial for maintaining pH and glucose level in blood.

(E) To Maintain Victims general Condition

In case of an unconscious victim, maximum danger is of upper respiratory infection. To avoid this risk of infection, the prophylactic antibiotic therapy must be given. Also management of hypothermia, intensive supportive treatment and good nursing care is required to maintain the general condition of victim.

INSECTICIDE POISONING

(A) Organophosphorus Compounds

The Compounds of this class include:

(a) Alkyl Phosphates: Hexaethyl Tetraphosphate (HETP), Tetraethyl Pyrophosphate (TEPP), Octamethyl pyrophosphoramide (OMPA) and malathion.

(b) Aryl phosphates Parathion (Folidol) and Diazinon (Tik - 20).

Symptoms	Fatal dose	Treatment
Poison first affects the smooth muscles and glands and then vital brain centres.	**HETP:** I.V., I.M. 160 mg Oral - 350 mg	1. Decontamination
Initially headache, malaise, constriction of chest and pin-point pupils.	**OWA:** IV., I.M. - 80 mg Oral - 175 mg	2. Artificial respiration. Positive pressure respiration. Tracheostomy if required.
After a few hours nausea, vomitting, diarrhoea, abdominal cramps, sweating, salivation and muscular twiching.	**TEPP:** I.M., I.V. - 45 mg Oral - 100 mg	Antidote therapy Atropine - 2 mg I.M. or I.V. every 15-30 min. to counteract muscarinic effects of Ach.
In severe poisoning, pulmonary oedema, coma, convulsions and death may result.	**Malathion:** 1 g **Parathion:** I.V., I.M. - 80 mg Oral - 150 mg **Diazinon:** 1 g orally	Cholinesterase reactivators therapy: Pralidoxime chloride, Pralidoxime iodide and pyridine aldoxy methiodate (PAM) in a dose of 1-2 g I.V. for adults. Repeated after every 12 hours.

(B) D.D.T

Symptoms	Fatal dose	Treatment
Oral route: Salivation, nausea, vomitting and abdominal pain		If ingested then material must be removed from G.I.T. by lavage and cathartics. Fats and oils should be avoided.
Contact: Irritation of eyes, nose, throat, blurred vision, pulmonary oedema, dermatitis. Nervous symptoms include hyper irritability, muscle spasms and tremors, convulsions, paralysis of limb muscles, collapse and death due to respiratory failure.	150 to 1000 mg per kg of body weight.	Adrenaline should not be used. Artificial respiration. If muscular twitching then give barbiturates or diazepam.

(C) Endrin

Symptoms	Fatal dose	Treatment
Vomitting, abdominal pain, convulsions, oozing of white froth from mouth and nostrils, dyspnoea, coma, respiratory failure and death.	6g.	Decontamination. Artificial respiration. Barbiturates to control convulsions. 10 ml 10% solution of calcium I.V. for every 6 hours.

(D) Napthalene

Symptoms	Fatal dose	Treatment
Acute nephritis, haemolytic anaemia, jaundice and optic neuritis. After ingestion it causes gastric irritation with nausea, vomitting and abdominal pain. Pains in urethra, bladder and kidney. Urine may be brown or black.	Approximately 2 g	Keep the patient warm. Stomach wash with warm water or saline. Use of magnesium sulphate to clear the bowels. Administer sodium bicarbonate to maintain the urine alkaline which prevents formation of acid haematin crystals.
Severe poisoning causes liver and kidney damage resulting in convulsions, cyanosis, coma and death. After inhalation it causes headache, nausea, vomitting, malaise, conjuctivitis, mental confusion and visual disturbance.		Blood transfusion may be necessary. Hydrocortisone for haemolysis.

(B) Heavy Metal Poisoning

Symptoms	Fatal dose	Treatment
1. Arsenic **Acute Poisoning:** Widespread damage to the capillaries. Severe gastroenteritis, dysphagia, epigastric and abdominal pain, vomitting, watery or blood diarrhoea, jaundice, oliguria, muscle cramps. Pale anxious face, sunken eyes, dilated pupils, rapid pulse, sighing respiration followed by convulsions, coma and death.	100-200 mg	Stomach wash with warm water. Freshly precipitated hydrated ferric oxide as antidote which forms harmless ferric arsenite. I.V. sodium thiosulphate 1 g in 10 ml sterile water every 4-6 hours for first day. I.M. Dimercaprol as specific antidote. **Dose:** 3 mg/kg body weight every 3 hours for first two days. Then 3 mg/kg body weight every 6 hours. On third day and then same dose every 12 hours till symptoms disappear. Morphine for controlling pain.
Chronic poisoning: Peripheral or optic neuritics, diarrhoea, conjuctivitis, pigmentation of skin, liver, cirrhosis and dependent oedema. It also causes palmer and plantar keratoses and carcinomas. A characteristic state of ill health appear. Four stages appear successively. **(i) Stage I :** Related with nutritional type anorexia, occasional vomitting, diarrhoea, easy fatiguability. **(ii) Stage II:** Catarrhal - conjuctivitis, running of eyes, running of nose, sense of fullness of head. **(iii) Stage III:** Skin rash, hyperkeratosis of foot, brittle nails, falling of hair. **(iv) Stage IV:** Related with CNS - Convulsions, Coma.	100-200 mg	1. Removal of patient from exposure. 2. I.V. sodium thiosulphate, 1 g in 10 ml sterile W.F.I. 2-3 times/week for many weeks. 3. Dimercaprol. Dose schedule same as acute poisoning.

2. Lead **Acute Poisoning:** Metallic taste, vomitting, colic pain in abdomen, constipation, black faeces, urine suppressed, lead encephalopathy Headeache loss of sleep, loss of vision, hallucination, delirium and convulsions. Acute haemolytic crisis may occur.		Stomach wash with 10% solution of magnesium sulphate followed with plain water. Bowel should be washed at regular intervals. Calcium Versenate (EDTA) or penicillamine should be used as antidote.
Chronic Poisoning: (Plumbism) Facial pallor, lead line (bluish-black line on the gums). Anaemia with punctuate basophillia (Presence of dark blue spots in cytoplasm of R.B.C.) constipation paralysis of muscles of wrist; Encephalopathy, Hypertension, Nephritis, Menstrual disorders, Abortion. **General symptoms:** Metallic taste, norexia, dyspepsia, headache, weakness, vertigo drowsiness.	0.5 g	Excretion of lead i.e. deleading by acidosis combination of EDTA and BAL is effective. EDTA 3 mg is mixed with saline and given by I.V. drip. BAL - 4 mg/kg body weight ever 4 hours.
3. Mercury **Acute Poisoning:** The main feature is metallic taste in mouth. The tongue, mouth become greyish white, nausea, vomit contains white mucus with blood. Cold skin, pale face, dilated pupils, shock, renal failure and liver damage.		Removal of poison by emetics or stomach wash with 5% solution of sodium formaldehyde sulfoxylate. Charcoal powder, 3-4 tablespoons with water. BAL in usual dose.
Chronic poisoning: Multiple neurological disorders such as shyness, irritability, tremors, loss of memory, loss of sleep, halucinations and insanity. This disorder is also called as "erethism". Excessive salivation with metallic taste is a peculiar symptom. Loosening of teeth with painful gums. Colitis, anemia, hypertension, renal failure. Mercuria lentis - discolouration of lens of eye due to deposition of mercury.		(i) Removal of patient from exposure. (ii) Promoting elimination of mercury by kidneys and bowels. (iii) Dimercaprol therapy for chelation. (iv) For excessive salivation – Dry extract of belladona 30 mg/ 3 times a day.

4. Copper: It is not poisonous in metallic state but some salts (e.g. copper sulphate) are poisonous. **Acute Poisoning:** Metallic taste with excessive salivation and thirst, abdominal pain diarrhoea. Vomit: Green or blue. Stools : Brown without blood. Urine: Like ink, containing albumin. **Chronic Poisoning:** Symptoms are similar to lead poisoning.	30 gm of copper sulphate	Same as mercury poisoning. 600 ml of potassium ferrocyanide in a glass of water to be given before performing gastric lavage. Same as for chronic mercury poisoning.

(C) Barbiturate Poisoning

Symptoms	Fatal dose	Treatment
Nausea, mental confusion, respiratory depression, drowsiness, deep sleep, hypotension, skin rash, muscle spasm, cyanotic face. Barbiturate automatism in few cases (patient takes more drug automatically forgetting that he has already taken a dose). Alternate contraction and relaxation of the pupil, hypotension. Decreased urine formation. Death occurs due to respiratory failure.	3-5 gm	1. Gastric lavage with potassium permangnate. 2. Artificial respiration 3. To elevate B.P. 2.5 mg Metarminol, I.V. 4. 5% glucose saline I.V. drip. 5. Coramine I.V. 5 ml 25% followed by 10 ml in 15 minutes and then 20 ml every 30 minutes till reflexes return. 6. Haemodialysis 7. Forced diuresis 8. Enema

(D) Narcotic Drugs Poisoning

Symptoms	Fatal dose	Treatment
I. Opium: The symptoms appear in three different stages. **(a) Excitement:** Pleasurable mental excitement with increase heart rate. **(b) Sopor:** Headache, giddiness, a sense of weight in limbs. Itching, cyanosis of face and lips and meiosis strong tendency for sleep. **(c) Narcosis:** Patient enters in to a deep coma, relaxation of muscles, loss of reflex, pinpoint pupils, hypotension lowered respiration, hypothermia frothing from mouth and finally death.	2 g or 200 mg or morphine	(1) In early stage, stomach wash with tepid water first and then with solution of potassium permanganate (2) Continue stomach wash till returned water is of pink colour. (3) Clear the intestine by enema. (4) Antagonist therapy 5-10 mg Nalorphine, I.V. every 15 minutes till dilation of pupil. (5) Naloxone 0.4-0.8 mg I.V. every 15 minutes. (6) For shock 1 lit. 5% glucose saline solution.

2. Cocaine: Euphoria, dysphagia, mydriass, dry mouth, numbness, heart rate increases, cyanosis sweating hallucinations, black tongue, nasal perforations. **3. Belladona alkaloids:** (Atropine) (Dhatura) Hyoscyamus. Dry mouth, bitter taste dysphagia, abdominal pain, hot dry skin, mydriasis, diplopia, vomitting, giddiness, delirium, fever, vision blurred, heart rate increased with increase in respiration.	1 g 125 mg or 15-30 mg Hyoscine	Gastric lavage with $KMnO_4$ or tannic acid. In local application, wash the skin with water. Artificial respiration. Cardiac stimulant therapy. Medicinal charcoal can also be employed. (1) Stomach wash with 5% tannic acid. (2) Neostigmine 2.5 mg I.V. every 3 hours. **OR** (3) Physostigmine 1-4 mg every 1-2 hours. (4) Sponging for raised body temperature. (5) For excitement-Diazempam 10 mg I.V.
4. Cannabis: Excitement followed by hallucinations, increased muscular movements, mental confusion, drowsiness. Mydriasis, deep sleep.	Charas - 2 g Ganja - 8 g Bhang - 10 g Per kg body weight	Gastric lavage, saline purgatives, I.V. fluids, hypodermic injection of strychnine. Artificial respiration.
5. Pethidine: Dry mouth, mydriasis, flushed face, tachycardia hyperthermia, drowsiness coma.	2 g	Gastric lavage, Coramine I.V., Symptomatic treatment.

QUESTIONS

1. Define the terms
   (a) Toxicology
   (b) Poison
   (c) Antidote
   (d) Chelating agent

2. Classify poisonous substances with examples.
3. Describe the basic principles of a general treatment for poisoning.
4. Give the different types of "antidotes" used in the treatment of poisoning with examples.
5. Give the doses for the following antidotes:
   (i) BAL
   (ii) Penicillamine
   (iii) EDTA
   (iv) Desferrioxamine
6. Give the symptoms and treatment for poisoning by:
   (i) Organophosphorus compounds
   (ii) D.D.T.
   (iii) Barbiturates
   (iv) Heavy metals
   (v) Narcotic drugs.
7. Give the composition, uses and dose of "Universal antidote".

***

9

DRUG DEPENDENCE AND ABUSE

The use of drugs for non-medical purposes is becoming increasingly common specially among the younger age groups of society. The indiscriminate use of drugs is becoming a serious public health and social problem.

Repeated administration of the drug causes habit and dependence. If habit forming drug is not made available to the patient, then withdrawal symptoms occur. These symptoms are psychic disturbances like headache, restlessness, emotional upset or physical disturbances like convulsions and vasomotor collapse.

The World Health Organization (WHO) Expert committee on Drug Dependence has given the definitions of the following terms as:

(1) Drug Dependence

"A state of psychic and also sometimes physical disturbances resulting from the interaction between living organisms and drugs showing behavioural and other responses that always include compulsion to take the drug in order to experience its psychic effects or to avoid discomfort. Tolerance may or may not be produced. A person may be dependent on one or more drugs. The two different types of drug dependence are:

(i) Physical dependence: In case of physical dependence, the tissues become adapted to the drug and if the drug is suddenly withdrawn, various abnormal reactions occur which are termed as abstinence syndrome or withdrawal symptoms. The physical dependence and withdrawal symptoms occur due to drug induced alterations at the cellular level with the prominent changes occurring in the CNS at all segmental levels. Physical dependence also leads to the development of tolerance. The withdrawal reactions are often severe depending on the drug and duration of use.

(ii) Psychologic (Psychic) dependence: The drug produces satisfaction and pleasure in such a way that requires further administration to maintain the sense of pleasure or to avoid discomfort. It denotes the compulsive need to experience a pleasurable drug reaction and person obtains the drug at any cost i.e. the craving for a particular drug. The term 'habituation' is often used interchangeably. It differs from physical dependence in that in psychologic dependence there are no serious withdrawal symptoms on sudden withdrawal of the drug which may endanger the life of the patient.

Addition: A condition in which there is both psychic and physical dependence. There is an overpowering desire to continuous take drugs, a tendency to increase the dose and high tendency to withdrawal symptoms.

Most of the drug used by addicts, particularly, effect CNS. e.g. opiates, barbiturates, alcohol. These drugs produce a feeling of well-being called euphoria.

The addicts continue taking drugs for the following reasons:

1. At first for its medicinal use.
2. To satisfy curiosity about the drug effect.
3. To have new thrilling or dangerous experiences.
4. To relax from stress and strain.
5. To escape from reality and have a dreamy state.

Experience achieved by the addict under the influence of drug is so impressive that he develops a craving for the drug and finds it difficult to give it up. Hence, the drug is called masterful drug. The exact mechanism of drug dependence is not known but change in cellular metabolism of CNS is an important factor in the development of drug dependence. The other systems may become tolerant to the drug but only CNS is capable of developing dependence.

Habituation: It is a pattern of repeated drug usage, although the actual physical need for the drug is minimal.

Comparison of Addiction and Habituation

No.	Drug Addiction	Drug Habituation
1.	It is a state of periodic or chronic intoxication produced by repeated consumption of a drug.	It is a condition resulting from repeated administration of a drug.
2.	An overpowering desire or need (compulsion) to continue taking the drug and obtain it by any means.	A desire (but not compulsion) to continue taking the drug for the sense of well-being that it produces.
3.	A tendency to increase the dose.	Little or no tendency to increase the dose.
4.	Effect of drug produces both psychological and physical dependence.	Effect of drug produces some degree of psychological dependence but no physical dependence and hence absence of abstinence syndrome.
5.	The effect is detrimental to the individual and to the society.	A detrimental effect, if any primarily on the individual.

Drug misuse: It refers to the improper use of medicines in a way that can lead to acute and chronic toxicity.

Drug abuse: It is the persistent or sporadic, excessive use of drugs, inconsistent with, or unrelated to medical practice. Drug abuse goes well beyond mere misuse of drugs.

Classification: The drugs of abuse are classified as under:

(1) CNS depressants: e.g. Alcohol, Barbiturates, Non-barbiturate, Sedatives and Tranquillizers.

(2) **CNS stimulants:** Amphetamine, Cocaine, Tobacco.

(3) **Narcotics:** Heroin, morphine, opium, codeine, pethidine, methadone.

(4) **Hallucinogens:** Marhihuana (Cannabis), LSD, mescaline, phencyclidine.

(5) **Volatile inhalants:** Benzene, Acetone, Petrol, Trichloroethylene.

CNS – depressants:

(1) Alcohol:

(a) Acute alcoholism: The enzyme alcohol dehydrogenase is responsible for metabolism of alcohol. It metabolises about 10 mg pure ethanol/hour. The features of acute alcoholism depend on the blood level.

Blood level mg/100 ml	Feature
20	Feeling of warmth and relaxation
30	Relief from anxiety
50	Inco-ordination, euphoria, speech mistakes
100	Ataxia
100-200	Vomitting, imbalance, vertigo
300	Stupor
400	Respiratory depression, coma.

Treatment: The treatment is supportive to maintain the respiration, blood pressure and body temperature. Until the ethanol is removed from the body by metabolism or haemodalysis. If intracranial, pressure is increased, administer hypertonic mannitol solution intravenously. Phenothiazine is used to control psychotic behaviour.

CNS stimulants should not be used as these may cause convulsions. Give artificial respiration and electrolytes for balance.

Chronic alcoholism: It results in development of tolerance and then physical dependence. The withdrawal of alcohol results in tremors, fits, anxiety, insomnia, confusion, G.I. disturbances like chronic gastritis, peptic ulcer, hepatitis, cirrhosis, pancreatitis. The abrupt termination after longer periods of alcohol abuse can lead to delirium tremens (fever, tremors, tachycardia, agitation, sweating, hallucinations and convulsions). It also results in myopathy, bone marrow suppression, and gout.

Treatment: It consists of counselling and attention to social and behavioural factors, supportive social interaction. (Alcoholics Anonymous), follow up. It also requires pharmacotherapy with antianxiety agents and aversion therapy using disulfiram.

Give Diazepam: 40 mg daily for 4 days
30 mg daily for 3 days
20 mg daily for 2 days
10 mg for 1 day

give intravenously (10 mg state then 5 mg every 5 minutes until calm) supplemented with haloperidol 2-4 mg every 4-6 hours.

Give high dose of Vitamin B-complex.

Chlormethiazole is an excellent sedative, anxiolytilc and anticonvulsant but has an addiction risk. Lorazepam is useful if there is hepatic dysfunction.

(2) Barbiturates: (Taken orally, I.V. or S.C.)

The chronic abuse of barbiturates results in drowsiness, ataxia, nystagmus, reduced quality and quantity of work, increased appetite, impaired motor co-ordination, confusion, emotional instability and poor judgement.

Withdrawal symptoms: Range from anxiety, confusion, insomnia, anorexia, panic attacks, tremors to delirium, disorientation, hallucinations and fits (sometimes status epilepticus).

Treatment :

(1) Gradual withdrawal of the drug by decreasing the dose over a period of three weeks.

(2) Psychotherapy is recommended.

(3) CNS - Stimulants : Amphetamine

Taken orally, intravenously or sniffed.

These drugs are widely abused for their CNS stimulant effect by students, atheletes, truck drives, executives, doctors and nurses. The therapeutic dose of amphetamine is 5 to 15 mg/day. It induces physical, dependence. Its acute administration results in excitement, euphoria, little need for sleep, anorexia, psychotic schizophrenia like reactions tachycardia arrhythmias, hypertension and fits. Cocaine when sniffed can lead to ischameic perforation of the nasal septum.

Withdrawal symptoms: Depression, fatigue, muscle, pain, hyperphagia, hypersomnia, lethargy.

Treatment:

(1) 8 mg of reboxetine per day is recommended for atleast 2 weeks. However, this drug is still in the trial stage.

(2) No other available treatment has been effective in the treatment of amphetamine withdrawal.

(4) Cocaine:

The chronic use of cocaine results in the following systemic effects.

(i) CVS: Myocardial infarction, arrhythmias.

(ii) CNS: Irritability, anxiety, hallucinations, insomnia, visual disturbances.

(iii) GIT: Nausea, weight loss, gangrene.

(iv) Urinogenital: Difficulty in erection and delay in orgasm in both sexes.

(v) Respiratory Perforation of nasal septum pulmonary oedema, rhinitus.

Treatment: Regular supportive therapy with tricyclic antidepressants and tranquilizer rugs. The vital functions of cardivoscular and respiratory system should be monitored.

(5) Narcotics:

e.g. *Morphine, opium, heroin, codeine* and *pethidine.*

The abuse of narcotics results in a syndrome constituting a drowsy and relaxed feeling, restlessness and excitements, pin point pupils, malnutrition, vitamin deficiency, thromboembolic complications, constipation, hepatitis, vasculitis, infection specially AIDS, pulmonary oedema, cardio-respiratory collapse and coma.

Withdrawal symptoms: Sudden withdrawal of opiates develops the following symptoms as below:

After 8 hours	:	Yawning, sweating, anxiety, tearing, rhinorrhoea.
20 hours	:	Gooseflesh, chills, sweating, panic.
24-48 hours	:	Nausea and vomitting, diarrhoea, fever, hypertension.
Upto 1 week	:	Muscle cramps
Upto several months	:	Insomnia

It is accompanied by craving for the drug.

Treatment: The symptoms can be suppressed by substitution of another narcotic for opiate e.g. Methadone - (20 mg in divided doses for first 3 days and then 10 mg for 3 days).

A newer compound, levo-alpha-acetylmethadol (LAAM) which is a longer acting drug is being used for narcotic addiction. This drug is superior to methadone, as it is not to be administered daily.

Naltrexone (Trexan) is another long acting antigonist used for treatment of narcotic addiction.

(6) Hallucinogens:

Hallucinogens are a group of naturally occurring compounds and synthetic compounds capable of producing profound distortion of reality, resulting in confusion, delirium, amnesia and loss of sense of direction, space and time.

Cannabis: Taken orally or smoked.

Products of cannabis sativa are available in two forms:

(i) Hashish: Resin obtained from flowering tops.

(ii) Marihuana: Chopped leaves and stalks. The other products are charas, bhang, ganja.

It produces psychic dependence only.

The effects reported after 1 minute of inhalation of adequate dose are : feeling of floating and drowsiness, increased sensitivity to external stimuli resulting in distorted perception of time, colour, music and distance, social relaxation, memory impairment for short term, hallucinations, incoordination, panic and delirium may recur after intoxication has worn off. There may be confusion, disorientation, and acute psychotic reactions.

The major psychoactive ingradient present in cannabis is delta-9-tetrahydrocannabinol (THC). Chronic abuse of cannabis results in mild dementia and personality changes.

Treatment: A quiet environment and reassuring attitude helps during acute psychotic phase, in the management of overdoses. The extreme agitation is best controlled by diazepam.

LSD: (Lysergic acid diethylamide) is the most potent hallucinogen currently available in the form of tablet, thin squares of gelatin or impregnated paper. The average effective oral dose is 25-50 mcg.

(7) Volatile inhalants

Volatile liquids are commonly placed on a handkerchief and inhaled. The effects produced are CNS excitation, dizziness, auditory or visual hallucinations, tinnitus, blurred vision, slurred speech and a staggering gait. The larger dose may result in unconsciousness, delirium, stupor, coma, cardiac arrest and death. Amyl nitrite inhalation has been abused as a sexual stimulant.

Treatment: It is similar to that of barbiturates. Oxygen and other supportive treatment is required.

QUESTIONS

1. Define drug dependence and explain its two types.
2. Define "Drug abuse". Give reasons for the drug abuse. Classify the drugs of abuse with examples.
3. Give the treatment for abuse of narcotics and chronic alcoholism.
4. What are hallucinogens? Give the effects of its abuse.
5. Differentiate between "Drug addiction" and "Habituation".

***

10

BIOAVAILABILITY OF DRUGS

After administration of drug into various body parts, the drug has to enter the blood stream to reach the site of action (target tissue). The total amount of administered drug does not reach the site of action but only a fraction of administered dose is effectively absorbed. So it is important to know the various processes by which absorption of drug takes place and the factors which govern the absorption of a drug.

For a desired effect of a drug, it must achieve minimum effective concentration at its site of action. The term 'Bioavailability' denotes the fraction of drug dose, that reaches the systemic circulation. Bioavailability of a drug is defined as the amount or percentage of drug that is absorbed from administered dosage form and reaches the systemic circulation after non-vascular administration. When the drug is administered intravenously, its bioavailability is 100.

PROCESS OF ABSORPTION

It is important to know the manner in which a drug is absorbed. The absorption of a drug may either be direct or indirect but it involves the passage of a drug across the cell membrane. This passage is governed by the lipid barrier present at the permeable membrane. The actual mechanism of absorption is a very complex phenomenon and is not yet understood thoroughly. The following mechanisms occur in the process of absorption.

(1) Passive diffusion: The term passive diffusion means that a drug or substance is transported across the cell membrane without utilizing the energy. It is also called as simple diffusion. The rate of transfer of a substance is proportional to the concentration gradient across cell membrane. The drug molecules penetrate the cell membrane either by way of a passage through aqueous pores in the membrane or by dissolving in the membrane substance. Both fat-soluble and water-soluble molecules of small size may cross the cell membrane by simple diffusion.

(2) Active transport: It is a specialized process requiring energy. This process is independent of the physical properties of the membrane. In this process, the carrier molecule combines with a drug molecule to form a complex on one side of the membrane. This complex then diffuses through the membrane and dissociates into carrier and drug molecules when it reaches the other side of the membrane. After this the carrier returns to the original side of the membrane to repeat the process.

The plasma concentration-time curves are process useful for studying bioavailability differences of drug administered in different dosage form but containing same amount of the drug. This helps in selection of type of dosage form for a specific drug.

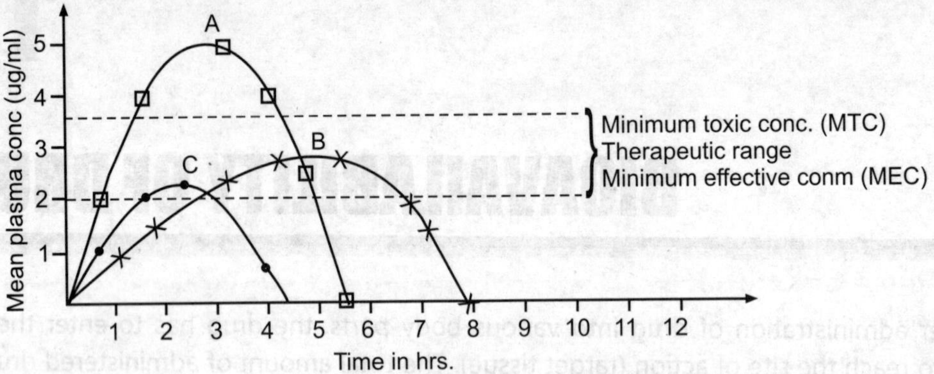

Fig. 10.1

From the curve, formulation 'A' would produce quick onset but short duration of action and formulation 'B' would produce the effect for much longer time. The formulation 'C' is therapeutically inactive because it would not achieve plasma concentration of drug for sufficient time. Also the formulation 'A' crosses the minimum toxic plasma concentration which may result in the toxicity of drug.

Bioequivalence : When the bioavailability of a drug from different formulations is the same, then it is called as bioequivalence.

FACTORS AFFECTING BIOAVAILABILITY OF DRUG

The factors affecting the bioavailability of drugs can be briefly summarized as follows:

(1) Physical state of drug: It is observed that liquids are better absorbed than solid medicaments. Also crystalloids are more readily absorbed than colloids and aqueous solutions are more quickly absorbed than oily solutions. Soluble medicaments like soluble insulin suspension is more readily absorbed than the insoluble protamine zinc insulin suspension.

(2) Particle size: It has been proved that small particle size is necessary for greater absorption of drugs from the gut. Smaller particle size provides greater surface area of a given weight of drug thus improving its absorption. Small particle size is useful in absorption of corticosteroids and antibiotics like chloramphenicol, griseofulvin and certain oral anticoagulants. Especially, for sparingly soluble drugs, particle size is the main factor affecting absorption. Thus, microfrine aspirin is better absorbed.

(3) Concentration: Higher concentration of drugs aids in better absorption of those drugs because most drugs are absorbed from the gut by passive diffusion mechanism.

(4) Dissolution rate: The absorption of a drug takes place only when the drug is in solution form. Hence, if the drug after disintegration (in case of tablet) gets dissolved quickly, then the absorption will be rapid and vice-versa.

(5) Absorbing surface: As compared to GI mucosa and pulmonary endothelium, skin is a poor absorbing surface. The absorption of a drug from floor of the mouth cavity (sublingual route) is faster. Thus, absorption of drugs from highly vascular membranes will also be rapid. Also drugs can be better absorbed from the small intestine than from the stomach. This is due to the large surface area of the intestine. Thus larger the surface area of absorbing surface, more will be the absorption.

(6) Functional integrity of GIT: Absorption of a drug from the G.I.T. can be effectively decreased by increased peristaltic activity. Thus anticholinergic drugs that reduce gut motility can affect absorption.

(7) Lipid solubility: If a drug is to be absorbed it has to pass through cell membranes of the mucous coat of G.I.T. and then into the circulation either via the blood capillaries or lymph channels. As cell membranes are lipid in nature, the degree and rate of absorption through them is dependent on the lipid solubility of the drug.

(8) Molecular weight: Drugs with high molecular weight need to be absorbed intact. They may get altered by enzymic action e.g. proteins will be broken down to respective amino acids. Thus, insulin undergoes enzymic breakdown in the gut and hence not absorbed effectively.

(9) Degree of ionization: Some substances like ethanol are unionized and others like acetylcholine are highly ionized in the gut. Majority of drugs are either weak acids or weak bases and at physiological pH (7.4) they exist partly in the unionized form and partly in the ionized form. The absorption process is usually proportional to the lipid solubility of the drug. The absorption of unionized form is greater because it is more lipid soluble than the ionized form.

(10) pH of drug: Acidic drugs are rapidly absorbed from stomach because in the acidic medium of stomach these remain in the unionized form.

e.g. *Salicylates* and *barbilurates.*

Basic drugs are not absorbed from the stomach. The alkaline environment of small intestine enhances the absorption of these drugs because these remain in the unionized form e.g. *Pethidine, Ephedrine.*

(11) Gastric emptying time: Rapid absorption occurs if the drug is given before meal. But certain irritant drugs like salcylates and iron salts are administered after food to minimize GI irritation.

Anticholinergic drugs which prolong gastric emptying time also decreases the absorption of drugs. Increased peristaltic movement reduces the drug absorption.

(12) Formulation: Formulation of the drugs also affects the absorption of drugs. It is observed that calcium and magnesium ions reduce the absorption of tetracyclines. Also the method of formulation influences the absorption of drug and thus determines its bioavailability.

Low degree of ionization, high lipid/water partition coefficient of non-ionized form and small molecular size of water soluble substances, all favour rapid absorption. Insoluble in both water and lipid prevent absorption e.g. Barium *sulphate.* Similarly insoluble precipitate formed in G.I.T. is not absorbed.

(13) First-pass metabolism: It means the biotransformation of the drugs during absorption through intestine and their transport through the liver in the portal circulation. It significantly reduces the percentage of oral dose that reaches systemic circulation. Drugs like propranolol, chlorpromazine are significantly metabolised in liver "first-pass effect".

When a drug passes through the liver for the first time, it is either destroyed in the G.I.T. or inactivated by the liver, then the sublingual route of drug administration can be used as the alternative route. In this case, the first-pass metabolism is avoided since the drug directly enters the systemic circulation. e.g. *Isoprenaline, Nitroglycerin.*

(14) Disease state of the gut: Absorption of drug may be affected by certain conditions like malabsorption, achlorhydria and cirrhosis of liver.

QUESTIONS

1. Define "Bioavailability". Discuss in brief the factors affecting it.
2. Describe various mechanisms of absorption of drugs.
3. Write a note on:
   (a) Active transport
   (b) First-pass metabolism
4. Define: (i) Bioequivalence (ii) Pinocytosis
5. How is bioavailability of drug determined?
6. Explain how the pH of drug and its ionization affects the bioavailability.

***

INDEX

***